Second Stage Labor Management:

Promotion of Evidence-Based Practice and a Collaborative Approach to Patient Care

By
Linda J. Mayberry, RN, PhD
Sylvia H. Wood, RN, MSN, CNM
Laura B. Strange, RN, MS
Lily Lee, RN, MSN, IBCLC
Darlene R. Heisler, RN, MSN
Kathryn Nielsen-Smith, MSN, CNM

Publication of this symposium was supported by an unrestricted education grant from Hill-Rom Company, Inc.

AWHONN
Association of Women's Health, Obstetric and Neonatal Nurses

About the Authors

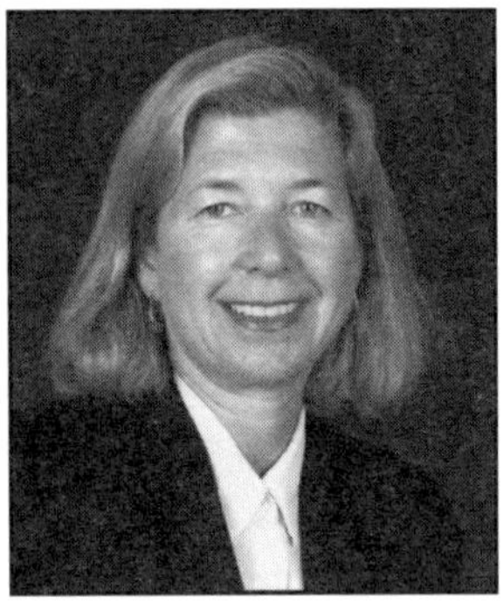

Linda J. Mayberry, RN, PhD is an associate professor for the Division of Nursing at New York University and an adjunct professor at Nell Hodgson Woodruff School of Nursing at Emory University, Atlanta Georgia. She served as the leader for AWHONN's Research Utilization Project on Second Stage Labor Management. Currently she is engaged in NIH/NINR research focused on stage labor management and epidural anesthesia. In 1999, Dr. Mayberry was awarded the prestigious "Award of Excellence in Research" from AWHONN.

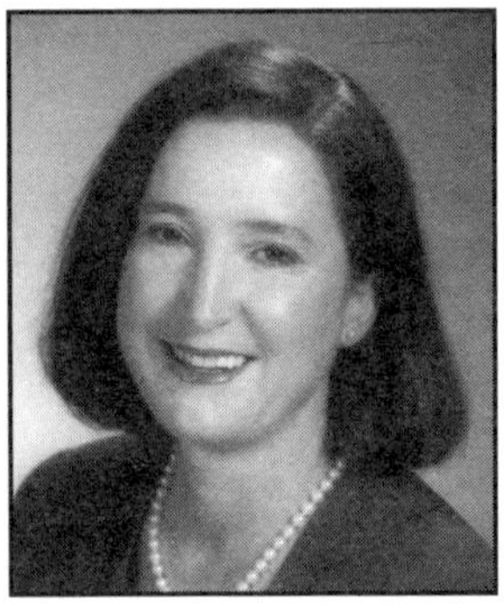

Sylvia H. Wood, RN, MSN, CNM is a certified nurse-midwife employed as an educator by Pacific Lutheran University, School of Nursing and as a practitioner by St. Joseph's Nurse-Midwifery Service, both in Tacoma, Washington. She served as the 1996 President of the Association of Women's Health, Obstetric and Neonatal Nurses (AWHONN). In 1997, Ms. Wood was awarded the prestigious "Distinguished Professional Service Award" from AWHONN. She was recently elected as a counselor for Psi-Chapter at Large of Sigma Theta Tau.

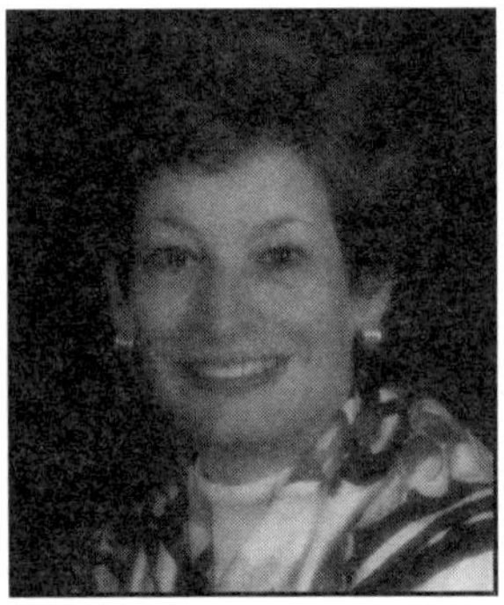

Laura B. Strange, RN, MS is an assistant professor at the Nell Hodgson Woodruff School of Nursing, Emory University, Atlanta, Georgia. She was a site coordinator for the second national AWHONN Research Utilization Project on Second Stage Labor Management. She is currently project director of a multi-site, NIH funded study evaluating nursing protocols for epiduralized women in labor. Laura is the Chair of the Atlanta Chapter, AWHONN, and has been accepted into the PhD program for nursing at Emory University for Fall, 1999.

About the Authors (continued)

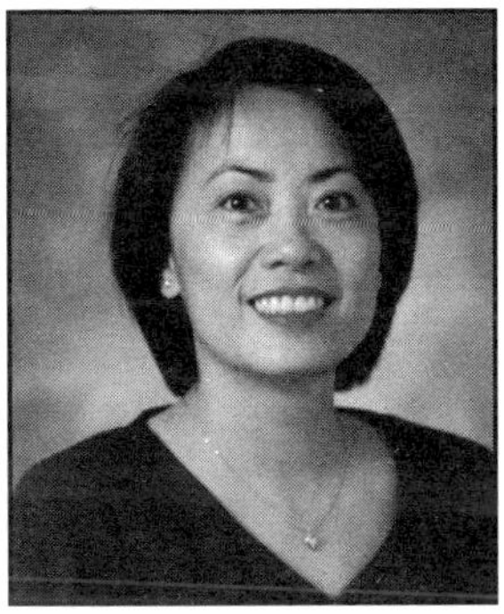

Lily Lee, RN, MSN, IBCLC earned a Bachelor of Nursing degree from the University of Manitoba and Master of Science in Nursing from the University of Texas at Austin. Lily is a perinatal clinical nurse specialist at the Royal Columbian Hospital in New Westminster, British Columbia, Canada, and an adjunct professor with School of Nursing, University of British Columbia. She was a site coordinator for AWHONN's Research Utilization Project on Second Stage Labor Management and continues to be actively involved in several research projects on labor and birth. An active AWHONN member since 1980 in both elected and appointed positions, she currently is the Communication Coordinator for the Canadian section of AWHONN.

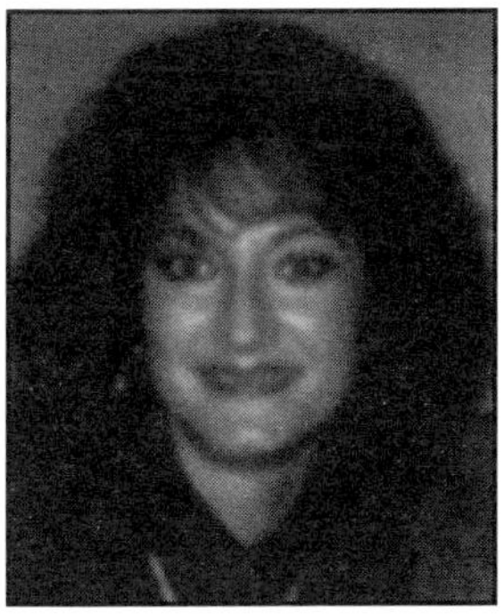

Darlene R. Heisler, RN, MSN began her career in OB-GYN nursing in 1975 when she graduated from Hamot Hospital School of Nursing with a Diploma in Nursing. She earned a Bachelor of Nursing from Loyola University in Chicago in 1981, and a Master of Science in Nursing in Maternal-Child Health in 1990. At present, she is a Level III Staff nurse in labor and delivery at Evanston's Women's Hospital, Evanston, IL and a student nurse midwife at Marquette University in Milwaukee, WI.

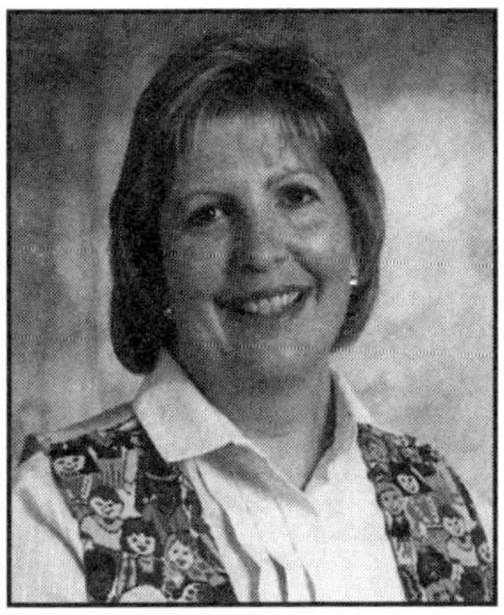

Kathryn (Kitty) Nielsen-Smith, MSN,CNM received a Bachelor of Nursing from William Jewel College. While completing her Master of Science in Nursing at the University of Missouri at Kansas City, she served as a site coordinator for the AWHONN Research Utilization Project on Second Stage Labor Management at St. Luke's Hospital of Kansas City. Since completing a post-Master's certificate in nurse-midwifery at the University of Missouri, Columbia, she is in private practice at The Clinic for Women, in Kansas City, Missouri. She is a member of AWHONN, ACNM, and Sigma Theta Tau.

Table of Contents

This Symposium was developed for AWHONN, the Association of Women's Health, Obstetric, and Neonatal Nurses, as an aid to nursing practice. It has been reviewed by nurses with expertise on this subject matter. AWHONN wishes to thank Linda J. Mayberry, RN, PhD, Sylvia H. Wood, RN, MSN, CNM, Laura B. Strange, RN, MS, Lily Lee, RN, MSN, IBCLC, Darlene R. Heisler, RN, MSN, and Kathryn Nielsen-Smith, MSN, CNM for their contribution in the development of this resource. This Symposium does not define a standard of care, nor is it intended to dictate an exclusive course of management. It presents general methods and techniques of practice that are currently acceptable and used by recognized authorities. Care of individual patients may depend on many individual factors as well as professional judgement. Symposium are reviewed every three years and revised if necessary. Publication should not be construed as excluding other acceptable methods of handling similar problems; appropriate variations and innovations that demonstrably improve the quality of patient care are to be encouraged rather than restricted.

Introduction and Purpose

Second stage labor management became a focus of obstetric researchers and clinicians during the 1990s. One reason for this focus has been the call for reduction in the cesarean section rate. Cesarean section rates in the U.S. escalated from 5% to 21% between 1970 and 1995 (Sachs, Kobelin, Castro, & Frigoletto, 1999). In 1990, the federal government set a goal to reduce cesarean section rates. A goal of 15% was set forth by the U. S. Department of Health and Human Services in the Healthy People 2000 report. Although most agree that 21% is too high, no evidence is available to support 15% as a target rate (Sachs, et al., 1999). Nonetheless, women who give birth via cesarean section have higher morbidity and mortality rates then women who deliver vaginally. Strategies to reduce the primary cesarean section rate have been identified (Flamm, Berwick, & Kabcenell, 1998), and one such strategy is to examine care practices during labor, including the second stage of labor.

Second stage labor management is complex. Many aspects of second stage labor management have been called into question, such as the practice of limiting the length of the second stage. Practices regarding positioning and pushing during the second stage also are being examined. Technologies, such as electronic fetal monitoring (EFM) and epidural analgesia that affect second stage labor management, should be examined as well. Integrated knowledge about all of these areas must be used to guide practice.

The purpose of this document is to improve the intrapartum care women receive in the hospital through promotion of evidence-based practice. Research related to the length of second stage labor; positioning; pushing techniques; and technologies, such as electronic fetal monitoring and regional analgesia are discussed. Much of the research discussed in this document was used to conduct the 1994-1995 Association of Women's Health, Obstetric and Neonatal Nursing (AWHONN) Research Utilization Project on Second Stage Labor Management. Findings from this project are presented, as are strategies for replication. Finally, improving collaboration among health care providers so that evidence-based practice can be achieved is addressed.

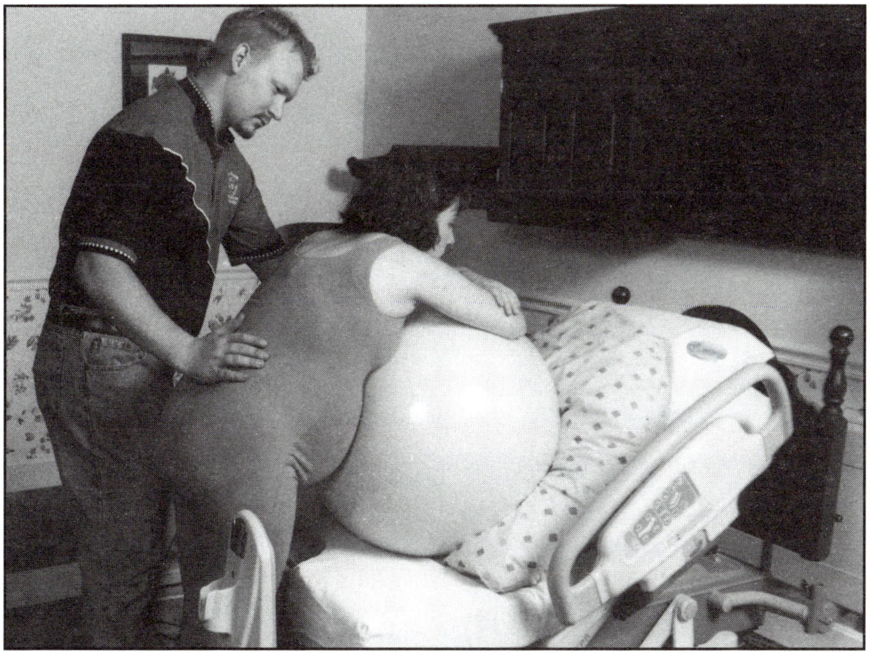

Laboring in an upright position using a birthing ball. Photograph compliments of Hill-Rom Company, Inc.

Length of Second Stage Labor

Efforts to limit the length of second stage labor have been documented since 1861 (Barnett & Humenick, 1982). The rationale was to decrease the risk of hypoxia to the fetus and thus improve neonatal outcomes. Endeavors to shorten the second stage led to practices such as encouraging directed, strong, sustained bearing down efforts with contractions and initiating pushing before the woman had an urge to push. No research has been documented to support these practices.

The rationale that shortening the second stage of labor improved neonatal outcomes was challenged more than 2 decades ago. Cohen (1977) studied the duration of the second stage among 4,430 nulliparous women and found no significant increase in the frequency of perinatal mortality or neonatal mortality when the second stage lasted longer. However, an increase in postpartum hemorrhage was found related to obstetric interventions used to limit the length of the second stage. Cohen's findings were supported by Menticoglou, Manning, Harman, and Morrison (1995). Their retrospective study examined the duration of second stage labor of 6,041 nulliparous women who delivered at a university teaching hospital during a 5-year period. No adverse outcomes were found in closely monitored patients, even when the second stage exceeded 5 hours in 2.7% of the patients.

The criteria for determining the time limits for the length of the second stage also have been challenged. Historically, Friedman's curve has been used to limit the duration of the second stage (Friedman, 1954). Albers, Schiff, and Gorwoda (1996) challenged the expectations for the length of labor as described in Friedman's 1954 study, "The Graphic Analysis of Labor," stating that no controls were used for variables such as Pitocin augmentation, caudal anesthesia, and forceps delivery. They studied the length of labor of a low-risk population of 1,473 women managed by certified nurse-midwives. Active labor without obstetric intervention lasted longer in 20% of their sample of healthy, low-risk women when compared with Friedman's curve. These study outcomes coupled with recommendations from the American College of Obstetricians and Gynecologists (ACOG, 1994) support efforts to de-emphasize a defined time limit (such as the "2-hour rule") for labor. According to ACOG, use of set time limits should be minimized because fetal monitoring techniques can identify a fetus who is not tolerating labor.

Positioning

Women have traditionally labored and delivered upright, either squatting or sitting using birthing chairs. The French obstetrician Francois Mauriceau (1637-1709) first introduced the recumbent position into obstetrics, believing it to be more convenient for the birth attendant and more comfortable for the laboring women (Dundes, 1987). The supine position for birth began to be used in the United States during the 19th century, coincident with the advent of medical care provided by obstetricians. It continues to be used in many hospitals (Shermer & Raines, 1997).

During the first stage of labor, upright positions, such as walking or standing, benefit the mother and the fetus. The decreased blood flow associated with horizontal positions may increase uterine muscle hypoxia and pain perception during contractions. Flynn, Kelly, Hollins, and Lynch, (1978) found that women who labored upright needed less analgesia. When women labor upright, gravity combines with fetal weight to exert an additional 10-35 mm Hg of pressure (Caldeyro-Barcia, 1979; Read, Miller, & Paul, 1981). Further, repeated clinical studies have shown that upright positions have a favorable effect on uterine contractility (Caldeyro-Barcia, 1979; Flynn et al., 1978; Read et al., 1981; Roberts, Mendez-Bauer, & Wodell, 1983). In a randomized, controlled trial, women who assumed upright positions (including squatting), experienced less pain and perineal trauma and fewer episiotomies than those delivering in supine positions (deJong et al., 1997). Higher fetal oxygen saturation during labor (Gupta, Brayshaw, & Lilford, 1989) and high pH and pO2 levels and lower pCO2 levels at birth (Caldeyro-Barcia, 1979) have been found in newborns of women who labored in upright positions, compared with those of women who labored in horizontal positions.

Traditional medical management includes using horizontal, semi-Fowler's and lithotomy positions during the second stage of labor, although these positions are disadvantageous for the mother and the fetus. These positions can slow fetal descent into the pelvis. A horizontal position centers maternal weight on the sacrum and coccyx, thereby restricting movement of the lower sacrum and adaptation of the pelvic structure to accommodate the fetus. Even in a semi-Fowler's position, the sacrum and coccyx encroach on the pelvic outlet, potentially interfering with fetal descent (Paciornik, 1990).

Nerve damage and lower extremity thrombosis may be related to poor alignment of the skeleton and pressure exerted by stirrups on the woman's lower extremities (Sloane, 1993). Other problems that may be associated with a horizontal position include an increased incidence of episiotomy and perineal lacerations (Hordnes & Bergsjo, 1993).

Squatting is the best position for second stage labor. The knees and hips are flexed, with the knees above the hips and the thighs pressed against the abdominal wall. In this position, the uterus elevates, directing the fetal presenting part toward the pelvic outlet so that fetal descent is enhanced. Golay, Vedam, and Sorger (1993) found that the mean length of second-stage labor was shortened by 23 minutes in primiparas and 13 minutes in multiparas who pushed while squatting, compared with women who pushed in a semi-recumbent position.

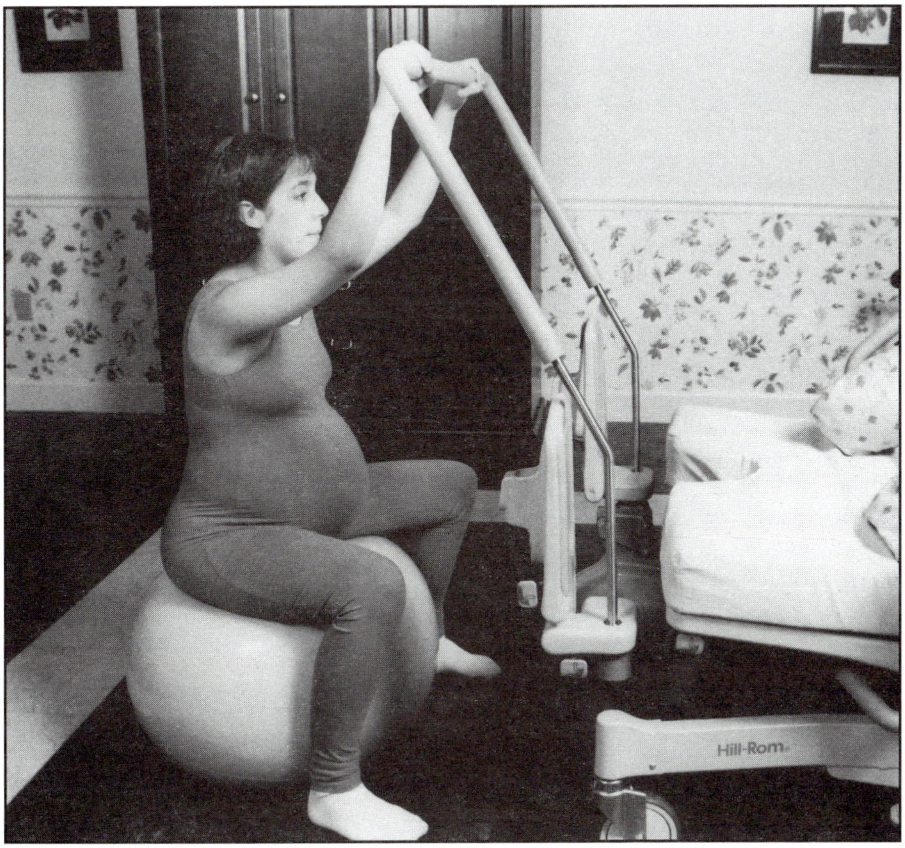

Using a birthing ball and squatting bar to simulate squatting position.
Photograph compliments of Hill-Rom Company, Inc.

Although squatting is the best position for pushing, women from westernized countries, such as the United States and Canada, typically have difficulty maintaining this position. In many non-western countries, squatting is a position used in everyday life while working or eating. Consequently, the thigh muscles are apt to be developed by daily use, and a squatting position for the second stage of labor may be easier to maintain. Assistance may be needed to help women to assume a variety of upright positions, including squatting, when delivering in our modern labor and delivery suites. If squatting is not an option, simulation of squatting may be achieved by sitting on a toilet or a birthing ball. Sitting in bed may be an option, although there is a tendency to slip into a semirecumbent position. When sitting, a women should be encouraged to maintain a forward thrust of her upper body as she would do if squatting (Shermer & Raines, 1997).

The use of continuous EFM influences many obstetric practices, including positioning. During the 1970s, continuous EFM was introduced as a technology with the potential to reduce neonatal morbidity and mortality. Today, continuous EFM prevails in the United States, often limiting the laboring woman's ambulation to a few feet near the monitor. Telemetry units have been developed to improve the woman's mobility, but are not available in every setting for every patient.

As researchers study the outcomes of continuous EFM, it has been shown that, for some populations, the outcomes are improved and for others outcomes are not affected. Researchers have questioned the efficacy of continuous EFM for low-risk populations (Leveno et al., 1986; Luthy et al., 1987; Rosen & Dickinson, 1993). Moreover, it has been suggested that continuous EFM increases the risk of operative intervention, liability for the physician and the hospital, and costs (Grimes, 1995; Sandmire, 1990). Thus, for low-risk women, the benefits of continuous EFM must be weighed against the side effects of limited mobility and unnecessary interventions.

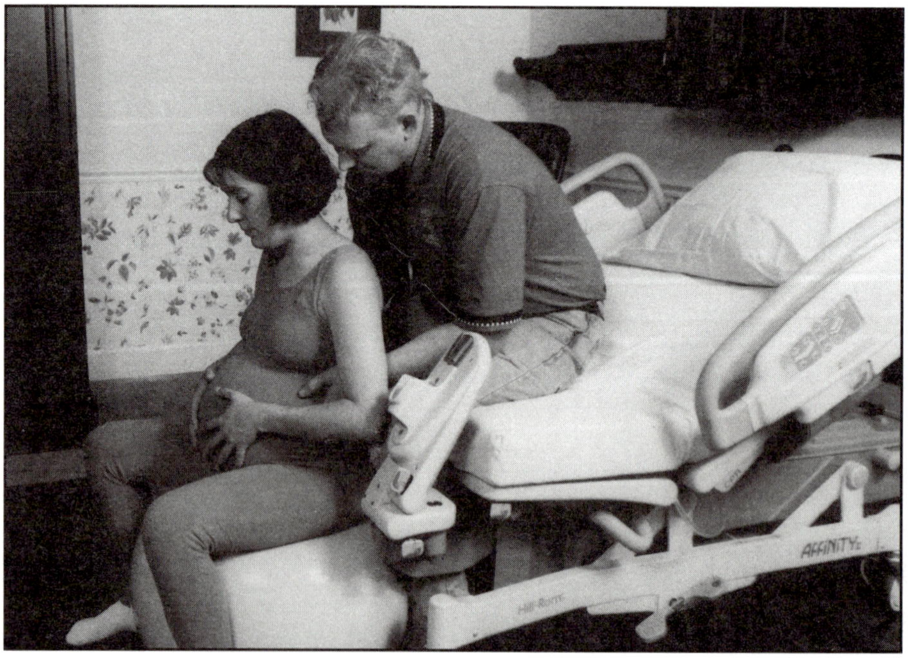

Laboring in an upright sitting position using a birthing ball.
Photograph compliments of Hill-Rom Company, Inc.

Pushing

Initiation of pushing and the technique used to push are practices that occur simultaneously. For clarity in this document, however, these two subjects are discussed separately. Both practices should be based on a response to Ferguson's reflex. Ferguson's reflex is the stimulation of nerve receptors in the pelvic floor in response to the pressure of the fetal head as it descends past the ischial spines.

Initiation of Pushing

To shorten the second stage of labor, the woman often is instructed to push when her cervix is fully dilated, whether she feels the urge to push or not. However, no research has been conducted to determine whether pushing at full dilation, regardless of station, shortens the length of second stage labor or enhances fetal descent.

Pushing for long periods of time may have negative outcomes. Long-term pelvic floor disorders have been at least partially attributable to obstetric management during labor (Handa, Harris, & Ostergard, 1996). The maternal consequences of unnecessarily prolonged bearing down may be increased fatigue during labor that can lead to a higher risk of cesarean delivery and, therefore, a lengthier postpartum recovery (Mayberry, Gennaro, Strange, Williams, & De, 1999). The fetal consequences of prolonged pushing may be decreased cerebral oxygenation and blood volume, resulting in fetal heart rate deceleration patterns (Aldrich et al., 1995; Holland & Smith, 1989; Schneider, Progler, Ziegler, & Huch, 1990).

Practitioners should encourage women to wait for spontaneous urges to bear down rather than relying on cervical dilation as the sole indicator for the onset of pushing (Roberts & Wooley, 1996). This practice is a physiologic approach to initiation of pushing based on stimulation of Ferguson's reflex. According to Roberts and Woolley (1996), this reflex usually is activated when the presenting part progresses to at least +1 station (descent past the ischial spines). At this point, involuntary bearing down pressures occur accompanied by exhalatory open glottis pushing by the mother. Sampselle and Hines (1999) reported that women who pushed spontaneously were less likely to have episiotomies and second- or third-degree perineal lacerations.

Exhalatory (Open Glottis) Bearing Down

Women are usually encouraged to push via directed, strong and sustained bearing down efforts with contractions. For example, the labor and delivery nurse or obstetrician often asks the woman to "hold your breath and push as hard [and as long] as you can" (Mayberry, 1994). Using this technique of pushing against a closed glottis (Valsalva's maneuver) has adverse hemodynamic effects on the mother. Prolonged breath holding causes an increase in intrathoracic and abdominal pressure, creating vasoconstriction and decreasing maternal cardiac output. As maternal blood flow is decreased, the volume of blood flow in the intervillous space is affected negatively. This situation can result in compromised perfusion in the fetus, with resulting changes in acid/base status. Non-reassuring fetal heart rate tracings are a sequela of this insult. (Barnett & Humenick, 1982; Caldeyro-Barcia, 1979; Holland & Smith, 1989; Sleep, Roberts, & Chalmers, 1989).

Researchers have suggested that exhalatory open glottis bearing down is the better pushing technique. The stimulation of Ferguson's reflex causes a physiologic, spontaneous bearing down by the woman. The woman involuntarily exhales (open glottis) and bears down three to five times during a contraction. Each push lasts 4-6 seconds (Roberts, Goldstein, Gruener, Maggio, & Mendez-Bauer, 1987). The woman will grunt and make other noises as she exhales and bears down. She needs no instruction to push in this manner, only encouragement and assurance that her effort and the accompanying sounds are normal. Paine and Dawkins-Tinker (1992) compared spontaneous pushing with Valsalva-type pushing and found no deleterious effects on umbilical cord gases with spontaneous pushing.

Epidural Analgesia

Epidural analgesia for pain management during the first and second stages of labor was introduced into the United States during the 1960s. It has become a popular and common pain management option for women in labor throughout the United States and Canada. Epidural anesthesia, a motor blockade used for operative deliveries, should be differentiated from epidural analgesia which affects pain, but does not necessitate the heavier motor blockade that can exclude use of upright positions during labor (Youngstrom, Baker, & Miller, 1996).

Researchers have found that epidural analgesia is correlated with a longer second stage and leads to a higher incidence of operative vaginal deliveries and cesarean sections (Dewan & Cohen, 1994; Ramin et al., 1995; Thorp et al., 1993). It is believed that women receiving epidural analgesia experience prolonged labor compared with non-anesthetized women, because relaxation of the pelvic floor musculature causes a delay in fetal head rotation. Factors that may contribute to the outcomes of epidural analgesia include the time in labor at which the epidural is administered (early versus late) and density of the epidural. Little research has been conducted regarding second stage labor management and epidural analgesia. However, the same principles related to upright positioning and pushing may apply.

Positioning and Epidural Analgesia

The benefits of upright positions for the first and second stages of labor were discussed in the section on positioning. Common obstetric management guidelines for women who receive epidural analgesia reinforce constricted mobility and non-upright positions. Obstetric epidural guidelines may include intravenous infusions, continuous EFM, confinement to bed, and analgesia dosage protocols that result in a heavy motor blockade (Shermer & Raines, 1997). Anticipation of potential side effects of epidural analgesia such as postural hypotension and lack of strength and control of the legs (Shermer & Raines, 1997) have led to these guidelines. These side effects vary according to the density of the epidural and analgesia dosage.

Researchers have studied differing analgesia dosage protocols that may reduce the side effects of epidurals and thus increase the opportunity for ambulation in labor, squatting during second stage, and ultimately effective pushing. Breen, Shapiro, Glass, Foster-Payne, and Oriol (1993) studied 130 women who received fentanyl alone or an ultra low-dose bupivacaine-epinphrine-fentanyl dosage. Both groups received adequate analgesia. Approximately 70% of the women in either group ambulated safely during labor.

> Recommendations from this study included criteria for determining the safety of ambulation with an epidural: (a) no obstetric or anesthetic contraindication to ambulate, (b) no postural hypotension, (c) normal leg strength, and (d) the ability to perform a satisfactory partial knee bend while standing. No woman with an epidural should ambulate unaccompanied.
> (Shermer & Raines, 1997, p.731)

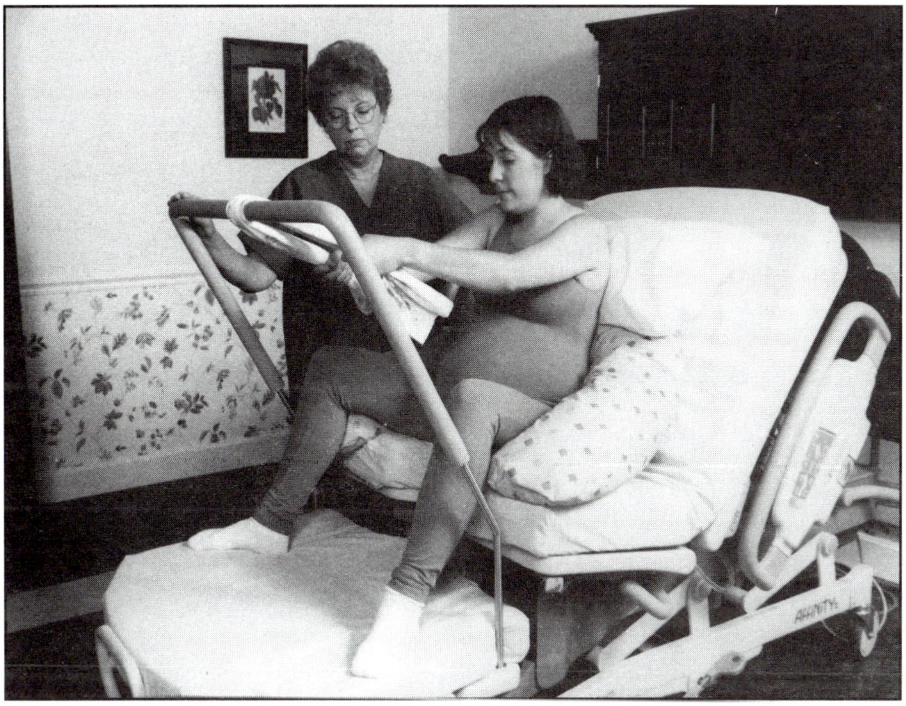

Modern birthing bed with squatting bar used to simulate upright position for pushing.
Photograph compliments of Hill-Rom Company, Inc.

Other strategies may be used to simulate upright positions for women with epidural analgesia who cannot squat for pushing. Birthing beds with squatting bars are available in some settings. When squatting bars are not available, an over-the-bed table covered with a pillow can be used for support.

> The foot portion of the birthing bed is lowered, and the table with pillow is positioned over the foot. The patient with head elevated high, is assisted to sit forward, grabbing the table to maintain a pelvic tilt while pushing. The table is held secure by the nurse or other assistant. Between pushes, the laboring woman can slouch a bit and lay her head on the pillow, maintaining the upright sitting posture. Without a birthing bed, the patient is assisted to a sitting position on the side of the bed, placing her feet on a cushioned stool or chair. The over-the-bed table is moved over the patient's lap and used in the same fashion as with the patient in a birthing bed. Another technique that can assist the woman to maintain a more upright posture is the "tug of war." Using a sheet or towel, the patient pulls and bears down during a contraction, while her "opponent" pulls in the opposite direction. (Shermer & Raines, 1997, p.732)

The advent of the intrathecal anesthetic techniques, in which women can more safely assume upright positions, will help to increase the use of such positions. Intrathecal narcotic analgesia (ITN) is a regional pain management method in which the narcotic is administered into the subarachnoid space instead of the epidural space. ITN is most effective during the first stage of labor. A few women are able to deliver with no additional analgesia or anesthesia during the second stage; however, some require further pain relief; such as a pudendal block or local anesthesia. Some anesthesia providers use a combined spinal/epidural technique so that epidural analgesia may be given if pain relief during the second stage of labor is needed (Shermer & Raines, 1997).

Smaller drug doses are used with ITN. Motor and sympathetic nerve blockades are not seen. The laboring women is able to ambulate and, depending on additional pain relief used during the second stage of labor, if any, may be able to push better than a woman with epidural analgesia.

Ropivacaine, as aminoamide local anesthetic, appears to offer advantages to the laboring woman. In comparisons of ropivacaine with bupivacaine, ropivacaine was found to provide comparable or enhanced pain relief without the intense motor block and risk of systemic toxicity associated with bupivacaine (Eddleston et al., 1996; McClure, 1996; Muir et al., 1997; Yun, Meadows, & Santos, 1998). Again, absence of a heavy motor block allows the laboring woman to assume more upright positions and affords greater control in terms of mobility.

Pushing and Epidural Analgesia

Women who receive epidural analgesia for labor often have difficulty pushing during the second stage. The decreased bearing down reflex and resulting decline in the efficiency of maternal pushing have been associated with the anesthetic effect, which itself prolongs labor and ultimately increases the risk for cesarean section (Dewan & Cohen, 1994; Lieberman et al., 1996; Philipsen & Jensen, 1989; Ramin et al., 1995; Thorp et al., 1993; and Wittels, 1991). The higher the density of the analgesic effect, the more likely the woman will not be able to push effectively. Attempts to avoid a prolonged labor may include promotion of strong, sustained, and directed Valsalva pushing by the laboring woman. In addition, women with epidural analgesia also are asked to push when they are completely dilated, regardless of station. With the fetal presenting part high and a diminished ability to bear down, women often push for long periods of time, sometimes several hours. The partial denervation of the pelvic floor that has been reported to occur following childbirth suggests the need to minimize unnecessarily prolonged pushing (Allen, Hosker, Smith, & Warrell, 1990). As stated in the section on pushing, prolonged sustained pushing sometimes leads to fetal hypoxia and nonreassuring fetal heart patterns, such as prolonged variable decelerations. Nonreassuring fetal heart rate patterns contribute to management decisions for operative vaginal deliveries and cesarean sections.

The practice of waiting for fetal descent before directing patients with epidural analgesia to push has been studied. Delayed pushing with epidural analgesia has been found to positively affect Apgar scores (Gleeson & Griffith, 1991; Manyonda, Shaw, & Drife, 1990; Maresh, Choong, & Beard, 1983; Vause, Congdon, & Thornton, 1998). Delayed pushing is also referred to as "laboring down", "passive pushing," or "rest and descend." Hansen and Clark (1996) studied women (N = 252) who received epidural anesthesia. Women who were allowed to rest for 1-2 hours at complete cervical dilation before beginning to push, experienced a slightly longer second stage. However, they also experienced shorter periods of pushing, a lower incidence of variable fetal heart rate decelerations, less fatigue, and Apgar scores equal to those who began pushing immediately after confirmation of complete dilation. Another randomized controlled study compared a group of women who began pushing at complete cervical dilation with a group of women who began pushing after a 1 hour rest period from the time of complete cervical dilation (Mayberry, Hammer, Kelly, True-Driver, & De, 1998). It was found that similar progress in descent was made (from 1-4 stations) during the 1st hour after complete cervical dilation. The mean difference in second stage labor duration between the two groups was only 14 minutes. Therefore, it may be prudent to re-evaluate management guidelines regarding the initiation of pushing, particularly when epidural analgesia is involved.

Evidence-Based Practice Through Research Utilization

Gennaro (1994) defined research utilization as "the process by which research knowledge is moved into the clinical arena" (p. 313). Research utilization may involve updating protocols for patient care or using a formal evaluation process to change clinical practice (Gennaro, 1994). Although the process is not always smooth, research utilization needs to be given priority if evidence-based practice is to be achieved.

Barriers and Facilitators of Research Utilization

When a change in practice is identified as necessary, the change agent(s) must be aware of the barriers and facilitators of research utilization. Through this awareness, the change agent can develop strategies to minimize the barriers and maximize the facilitators.

Barriers

In a national survey, various barriers to research utilization were identified and categorized (Funk, Champagne, Tornquist, & Wiese, 1995). Nurses reported that the quality of research affects the credibility of the recommendations. Specific concerns included studies with faulty research designs, conflicting outcomes, and failure of studies to be replicated or replicable. Nurses also commented on the difficulty of finding relevant clinical research with clear implications for practice. Institutional barriers also affected nurses' efforts to implement research into practice. Inadequate staffing frequently forces nurses into a survival mode so that the priority is just to get the job done. Nurses stated that feelings of powerlessness because of a lack of support from physicians and administrators impede innovative practice. Other barriers to research utilization are nurses' isolation from research activities and the inability to determine when recommendations are ready for implementation.

Facilitators

The ultimate goal of research and research utilization is to improve patient care. Researchers need to continually assess the readiness of their findings for application to clinical practice. Research utilization by nurses and physicians will be enhanced if reports are written clearly, with specific statements as to the interpretation of findings and applications to various settings. Criteria for nurses to use in evaluating whether research findings are ready for clinical application include the following (Lindsey, 1991):

1. *Significance.* Will meaningful improvement in the quality of care result if the recommendation is implemented?
2. *Scientific merit.* Is there evidence of scientific rigor in the study design, selections of sampling techniques, and analysis of the findings? Are the findings credible?
3. *Replication.* Has the study or elements of the study been repeated in other locations with other populations? Do the outcomes lend themselves to generalization?
4. *Transformation.* Are the findings from the study reported so that implications for practice are clear?
5. *Utility.* Do the conclusions provide a solution to a clinical problem?
6. *Applicability.* Is the clinical population and environment similar to the one studied?
7. *Feasibility.* Is there a cost/benefit advantage to implementing the findings?

The best clinical care settings are ones that promote inquiry and critical thinking. The administrators of a health care setting set the tone for the organization and should support and encourage research utilization. Providing leadership by example through targeted participation in the process and setting expectations for research utilization as a part of staff responsibilities will facilitate progress toward practice changes. Exposure to research by both administration and staff is essential and should include the availability of journals appropriate to the health care setting and access to literature searches.

Dialogue must occur between researchers and clinicians. Such dialogue is essential to achieving evidence-based practice by strengthening both the process for introducing new practices and the decisions made surrounding the need for new research. Nurses with research education and advanced practice nurses can jointly review studies and determine how they can be implemented in a particular setting. Collaboration with physicians and other health care providers is key, and multidisciplinary task forces may be formed to discuss specific practices (Funk et al., 1995). Internet resources, such as the Perinatal Nursing Discussion List and other Internet list serves provide forums for framing new ideas related to practice issues and for analyzing research outcomes and implementation strategies.

AWHONN's Research Utilization Project on Second Stage Labor Management

Research Utilization Priorities

Research utilization has been discussed in the nursing literature since the 1970s (Funk et al., 1995). One way to facilitate research utilization has been for nursing associations to conduct large, multisite projects involving their members as resources. AWHONN was one of the first nursing organizations to focus on the need to evaluate the process of research utilization. In 1990, AWHONN's Committee on Research convened a panel of nurse experts in obstetric, neonatal and women's health to identify "areas in which a sufficient base exists to guide implementation and evaluation of changes in clinical practice" (Gennaro, 1994, p. 316). (See Table 1.) The first AWHONN national research utilization project focused on improving neonatal thermoregulation. The project involved moving low birth weight infants from isolettes to open cribs at nine hospitals in the United States (Medoff-Cooper, 1994). The second project was based on two of the maternity nursing priorities:

- Use of upright versus recumbent positions during second stage labor to reduce fetal compromise and maternal pain
- Use of exhalatory versus sustained bearing down during second stage labor to reduce abnormal fetal heart rate patterns and low Apgar scores (Mayberry & Strange, 1997).

A smaller pilot project on the management of second stage labor had been conducted at three hospitals by members in former AWHONN District IX (Mayberry, Wood, & Held, 1993). This pilot project was expanded in AWHONN's second research utilization project to include 40 hospitals; 38 in the United States and two in Canada. More than 3,000 nurses participated in that process.

Process for AWHONN's Research Utilization on Second Stage Labor Management

Project Development

With the priorities identified, a literature search was conducted. "A synthesis of the extant research (Chalmers, Enkin, & Keirse, 1989) and of more than 50 articles on management of the second stage of labor were used to develop the practice "guidelines" in the form of a project protocol (Mayberry & Strange, 1997, p. 701) for second stage labor (see Table 2).

Next, sites and site coordinators were recruited through an announcement in AWHONN's newsletter, *The Voice.* Criteria for site selection included a letter of support from the institution to participate and an adequate number of deliveries at the site to ensure timely data collection. In addition, site coordinators sent a statement of intent to attend the orientation workshop held in July 1994 in Washington, DC (Mayberry & Strange, 1997).

At the orientation workshop, the project directors familiarized the site coordinators with research utilization concepts, the research related to second stage labor management, the project practice protocol, and the research-based guidelines (Table 2). Obligations of site coordinators were discussed, and the project structure and time lines for each phase of the project were outlined. Data collection tools were distributed, and questions about data collection were clarified (Mayberry & Strange, 1997). In addition, each site received a video to assist with educating staff nurses about the project guidelines. "The video contained information on second-stage labor research and a discussion of the issues and controversies surrounding nursing care management [Executive Communications, Inc., 1993]" (Mayberry & Strange, 1997, p. 703).

Table 1

Research Utilization Project Areas

Maternity Nursing

1. Identification of abused women through the routine use of screening questions.
2. Promotion of breastfeeding by modeling the home experience in the hospital.
3. Use of upright versus recumbent position during second stage labor to reduce fetal compromise and maternal pain.
4. Exhalatory versus sustained bearing down during second stage labor to reduce abnormal FHR patterns and low Apgar scores.
5. Use of antacids and dietary fiber in pregnancy.
6. Decreased use of pharmacologic analgesia in childbirth.
7. Reducing smoking during pregnancy through patient education programs.
8. Improving parental knowledge and skills about behavioral capabilities of newborn.
9. Reduction of depression and anxiety in bereaved parents through enhanced care strategies.
10. Practices to abandon, including:
    - Leaving women unattended in labor
    - Failure to include women in decision-making
    - Routine episiotomy
    - Advising restriction of weight gain.

Women's Health Nursing

1. Motivating women to initiate and maintain regular breast self-examination in conjunction with a regular program of clinical examination and mammography.
2. Promotion of pelvic muscle strengthening for mild and moderate stress urinary incontinence.
3. Preparation of mother-daughter dyads for menarche.
4. Preparation of women for menopause as a normal and healthy transition.
5. Use of both psychologic and physical examination components to routinely screen women for emotional, sexual, or physical abuse.

Neonatal Nursing

1. Use of comfort measures, such as non-nutritive sucking during or in anticipation of stressful procedures.
2. Removal of barriers to successful breastfeeding; improving breastfeeding success in preterm infants.
3. Improving skin integrity of low-birth-weight premature infants.
4. Improving thermoregulation of infants.
5. Reducing physiologic sequelae of infant suctioning.
6. Use of findings that infants do feel pain.
7. Use of telephone follow-up services, especially for high-risk infants and families.

These topics were identified by NAACOG's Research Utilization Task Force (1990) as areas in which a sufficient base exists to guide implementation and evaluation of changes in clinical practice. Topics for research utilization projects are not limited to those on this list.

Note: From "Research Utilization: An Overview," by S. Gennaro, 1994, *Journal of Obstetric, Gynecologic, and Neonatal Nursing, 23,* p. 316. Copyright 1994 by the Association of Women's Health, Obstetric and Neonatal Nurses. Reprinted with permission.

Table 2

Purpose: To apply research-based knowledge to the clinical practice of management of the second stage of labor. The goals are: (a) to assist in promoting the birth of the non-compromised fetus by minimizing negative maternal hemodynamic changes caused by inappropriate positions and pushing techniques and (b) to minimize maternal fatigue.

Positions for Second Stage

Practice	Rationale
1. All pregnant women should receive information prenatally on the benefits of upright positions for second stage prior to labor, which include a decrease in the duration and pain of labor as well as increase in the intensity of contractions.	1. Prenatal education can prepare women to take an active role in their labor and encourage practice of pushing positions second such as squatting (Cosner & deJong,1993; Liu, 1994; McKay, 1984).
2. Encourage the pregnant woman to try different positions throughout the second stage. Assist patients to turn side to side, at least every 30 minutes-1 hour if epidural in place.	2. No single position is appropriate for all labors. Varying positions can assist the fetus to maneuver down and out of the pelvis (Aderhold & Roberts, 1991; Holland & Smith, 1989; McKay, 1981).
3. Supine positions, such as lithotomy should be discouraged. (Refers to flat on back lithotomy position – not a semirecumbent/lithotomy position).	3. The lithotomy position causes compression of the inferior vena cava, aorta, and iliac arteries by pressure of the uterus against the mother's spine (Humphrey, Hounslow, Morgan, & Wood, 1973; Johnson, Johnson, & Gupta, 1991).
4. Suggested positions should include squatting, semirecumbent, standing, and upright kneeling. (Semirecumbent for patients with epidurals or side lying).	4. Increased intra-abdominal pressure can be generated in these positions because of increased efficiency of abdominal muscle contractions in addition to the force of visceral weight (Gardosi, Sylvester, & Lynch, 1989; Golay, Vedam, & Sorger, 1993; Roberts, 1980; Russell, 1982).
5. Squatting should be encouraged, especially for women with narrow pevic outlets and/or large fetuses. (No epidural patients.)	5. During a squat, both the anteroposterior and transverse diameters of the pelvic outlet increase 1-2 cm (Johnson, Johnson, & Gupta, 1991; Russell, 1982). Also, the pressure of the mother's thighs against her abdomen increases intra-abdominal pressure (McKay, 1984; Roberts, 1980).
6. The mother should be encouraged to lean forward and maintain a pelvic tilt with contractions during the first part of the second stage. (No epidural patients.)	6. Leaning forward will encourage the fetus to keep from resting on the sacral vertebrae, which can misalign the fetus' head and prevent it from entering the inlet (Davies & Renning, 1964; McKay, 1984). A pelvic tilt mobilizes the sacrum, enabling the fetus to rotate during its descent (Simkin, 1982).

Table 2 (continued)
Pushing Technique

Practice	Rationale
1. Review realistic expectations and sensations of second stage early in labor as well as at the onset of second stage.	1. Learning about the range of emotions and effort involved in second stage will assist the pregnant woman to prepare for the work and the sensations of second stage (McKay, Barrows, & Roberts, 1990).
2. Encourage spontaneous bearing down. If the fetal head has not descended low enough in the pelvis to stimulate Ferguson's reflex (stretch receptors in the pelvic floor), allow the mother to rest until she feels the urge to push.	2. Refraining from instructing a mother to begin pushing prior to the time she feels the urge to push minimizes maternal fatigue (Benyon, 1957; Roberts, Goldstein, Gruener, Maggio, & Mendez-Bauer, 1987).
3. Consider fetal station and position in addition to dilation in determining a woman's readiness for pushing.	3. Involuntary bearing down may be encouraged if fetal station is favorable (0 to 1+) as well as fetal position (OT to OA) regardless of a cervix which is dilated less than 10 cm (8-9 cm, soft and retracting) (Roberts, Goldstein, Gruener, Maggio, & Mendez-Bauer, 1987).
4. Discourage prolonged maternal breath holding (greater than 6-8 seconds) during pushing (4 or more pushing efforts per contraction).	4. Breath holding invloves the Valsalva maneuver: increased intrathoracic pressure due to a closed glottis causes a decrease in cardiac output and blood pressure. The fall in pressure causes a decrease in placental perfusion, causing fetal hypoxia (Caldeyro-Barcia, 1979).
5. Support rather than direct the woman's involuntary pushing efforts. These efforts may include grunting, groaning, exhaling during the push and/or breath holding less than 6 seconds.	5. Spontaneous, involuntary bearing down efforts match the intensity of each contraction. An open glottis, as seen with grunting and exhale pushing, avoids the Valsalva maneuver and has physiological benefits for both the mother and baby (McKay & Roberts, 1990; Roberts, Goldstein, Grueder, Maggio, & Mendez-Bauer, 1987).
6. Validate normalcy of sensations and sounds the mother is voicing.	6. Mothers and caregivers perceive low pitched groaning, sighing, and moaning to be sounds of tension release which may assist her in coping with the pain of second stage (McKay & Roberts, 1990).

Note: This protocol does not define a standard of care nor is it intended to dictate an exclusive course of management. It presents methods and techniques of practice that are currently acceptable and supported by research. The protocol should not be construed as excluding other acceptable methods of handling the second stage of labor or innovations that demonstrably improve the quality of patient care.

Note: From "Strategies for Designing a Research Utilization Project with Labor and Delivery Nurses," by L.J. Mayberry and L.B. Strange, 1997, *Journal of Obstetric, Gynecologic, and Neonatal Nursing, 26,* pp. 702-703.

This phase lasted 3 months. The site coordinators used this time to develop formal and informal support for starting the research utilization project on their labor and delivery units (Mayberry & Strange, 1997). Support from all levels of administration is important to research utilization. In general, the site coordinators started by presenting the project to the administrators or managers of the labor and delivery unit. Next, they sought support from department administrators, such as clinical directors of nursing and chairs of obstetrics. Finally, requests for support were addressed at the institutional level, such as nursing research committees, institutional research committees, or institutional human subjects review boards (IRBs) (Niesen & Quirk, 1997).

Site coordinators reported that challenges encountered during this phase generally were with the research committees, IRBs, or professionals outside of nursing. Apparently, the reason for the challenges stemmed from confusion among these groups about the difference between research and research utilization (Niesen & Quirk, 1997). Research utilization is a nursing term and had to be explained to committee members and other professionals outside of nursing. Once an understanding of research utilization was achieved, the project generally was approved as a quality assurance or continuous quality improvement project (Niesen & Quirk, 1997).

During this phase, three sets of data were collected before introducing the practice guidelines. Demographic surveys were completed by the site coordinators. Common beliefs and practices questionnaires were completed by staff nurses. One hundred Pre-Protocol Patient Data Forms provided baseline data before the protocol was introduced on the labor and delivery units (Mayberry & Strange, 1997).

This phase lasted two months. Each site coordinator designed a plan for guideline introduction and education of staff. Table 3 lists the 18 methods used by site coordinators (Niesen & Quirk, 1997). As previously stated, a video was provided to each site containing information on second stage labor research and a discussion of the issues and controversies surrounding nursing care management that was produced by Executive Communications, Inc., (1993) in collaboration with AWHONN (Mayberry & Strange, 1997). "Variety, humor, and a high degree of visibility were key factors in the successful introduction of the project protocol to nurses" (Niesen & Quirk, 1997, p. 712).

Sustaining the use of the guidelines once introduced was important. Site coordinators knew their colleagues best and were allowed flexibility for staff development and motivation (Niesen & Quirk, 1997). Presence of the site coordinators on the units was used as a motivator to the staff to remember to use the guidelines, to provide immediate recognition of staff working within the guidelines, and to provide opportunity to answer questions and problem solve (Niesen & Quirk, 1997). Other nurses were recruited to assist with motivation and champion the project (Niesen & Quirk, 1997).

Because second stage labor management may overlap with the domains of other health care professionals, collaboration was sought with obstetricians, anesthesiologists, family medicine physicians, and residents. Although most of these physicians were introduced to the guidelines during the first phase, site coordinators continued to obtain support for the project during the second phase and used various methods, such as follow-up letters with the guidelines attached, presentation of the guidelines at physician staff meetings, and one-on-one meetings with physicians. Some physicians questioned the research base used to develop the guidelines. Site coordinators viewed these occasions as a chance for further discussion and collaboration using research articles available on the unit (Niesen & Quirk, 1997). The site coordinators often sought support from the doctorally prepared project directors when the research needed to be discussed. At some sites, second stage labor management was viewed as primarily the domain of the nurse, because obstetricians were consulted only when needed or for delivery.

The nurses at these sites did not seek as much collaboration with physicians (Niesen & Quirk, 1997). At the end of phase 2, site coordinators reported their observations and insights about events that occurred during the first two phases (Mayberry & Strange, 1997).

Phase 3 — Protocol Implementation/Evaluation

This phase lasted approximately 3 months. During the first month, the protocol was implemented on the units. Next, 100 Post-Protocol Patient Data Forms were completed by the staff nurses participating in the project. The Post-Implementation Staff Summary was completed by the site coordinators and included their observations of medical and nursing staff reactions to implementation, clinical issues raised during this time, and results of individual staff nurse interviews. In addition, site coordinators completed a Protocol Assessment Form, which included a scaled assessment of the degree and frequency that each practice component in the guideline was met by the nursing staff (Mayberry & Strange, 1997). These data sets helped the site coordinator and nursing staff to identify patient care and professional issues associated with trying out the guidelines.

Table 3

Methods Used to Introduce the Second Stage Research Utilization Project and Protocol to Labor and Delivery Nurses

1. Informal inservice meeting
2. Staff meeting presentations
3. One to one education
4. AWHONN video
5. Distribution of protocol
6. Notebooks with articles
7. Self-learning packets
8. Memos/letters
9. Newsletters
10. Unit communications notebook
11. Posters
12. Fliers with key points of protocol
13. Journal club
14. Project implementation teams
15. Unit nurse cheerleaders
16. Creation of research utilization video
17. Research utilization pin worn by nurses

Note: From "The Process for Initiating Practice Changes in the Intrapartum: Findings from a Multisite Research Utilization Project," by K.M. Niesen and A.G. Quirk, 1997, *Journal of Obstetric, Gynecologic, and Neonatal Nursing, 26,* p. 709-717. Copyright 1997 by the Association of Women's Health, Obstetric and Neonatal Nurses. Reprinted with permission.

Phase 4 — Dissemination

This phase began in June 1995 and is continuing. Preliminary findings on the process issues of this research utilization project were presented by the project directors at the 1995 AWHONN National Meeting in Nashville, TN. Site coordinators presented their findings and experiences. They also offered consultation to nearby hospitals (Mayberry & Strange, 1997). Four articles regarding the project were published in *JOGNN* in 1997. Work on a clinical practice guideline for second stage labor management has begun as part of AWHONN's evidence-based practice program and is to be published in the year 2000.

Replicating the Research Utilization Project

Development of a Low-Risk Protocol for Second Stage Labor Management

Most institutions that provide obstetric care have guidelines outlining the management of care for high-risk patients or those at risk for poor obstetric outcomes. However, guidelines seldom exist to promote optimal care for the low-risk patients who make up the majority of the obstetric population. Without such guidelines in place, low-risk patients often are placed in the same care category as their high-risk counterparts. Underlying this approach seems to be the belief that the more intensive monitoring and medical interventions used to benefit high-risk patients will benefit, or at least not harm, those who are not. Based on the evidence presented in this symposia, this is not the case.

One of the first steps in implementing new guidelines for patient care is to develop a comprehensive protocol that can be evaluated. It is recommended that the guidelines within the second stage labor management protocol include the practices used in AWHONN's research utilization project on second stage labor management (see Table 2). The current authors recommend that the following four elements, which are evidence-based, be considered for inclusion:

1. **Maternal/fetal condition should be used to determine the length of second stage labor.** The evidence for this element was discussed in the previous section on the *length of second stage labor.*

2. **Continuous EFM should not be used routinely for low-risk patients.** Abandoning the practice of routine continuous EFM was put forth by AWHONN's Committe on Research in 1990 (Gennaro, 1994) (See Table 1). *Fetal Auscultation,* another symposia in this series, may be of interest to nurses working to incorporate auscultation protocols into their health care setting.

3. **Use of upright positioning should be individually assessed when women receive epidural analgesia.** The protocol for the Second Stage Labor Management RU project was developed in the early 1990's. At that time a more conservative stance was delineated related to upright positioning for women who received epidural analgesia because of the lack of available research findings (see Table 2, specifically practices #5 and #6). Although research findings still are limited, the combination of subsequent RU project findings and more recent published research findings, suggest that the more prevalent use of low-dose epidurals will allow the increased use of upright positioning. Therefore, it is now recommended that decisions about upright positioning for women who received epidural analgesia be made by an individual assessment in collaboration with the anesthesiologist, nurse, and the woman in labor.

4. **All patients should be provided support during labor.** AWHONN's Committee on Research accepted the contention that the practice of "leaving women alone to labor" be abandoned (Gennaro, 1994, p. 316) (See Table 1). Researchers have demonstrated the positive effects of continuous support in labor (Enkin, Keirse, Renfrew, & Neilson, 1993; Hodnett & Osborn, 1989). A meta-analysis by Hodnett (1996) examined labor support and provided evidence supporting the effectiveness of professional labor support. Women had shorter labors, required less analgesia or anesthesia and had fewer operative vaginal deliveries and cesarean sections when additional labor support was provided by doulas. A meta-analysis by Zhang, Bernasko, Leybovich, Fahs, and Hatch (1996) examined continuous labor support among young, low-income, primiparous women. The group that received doula support had twice as many spontaneous vaginal births, one-half the use of oxytocin and forceps, and one-half the incidence of cesarean section than the group that had no doula support. As these data are disseminated, particularly in the lay media,

consumer interest in doulas is expected to increase. According to Jennifer Nunn of Doulas of North American (DONA), inquiries from consumers for doula services amount to more than 199 per month from around the country (personal communication, April 1997). Requests from individuals inquiring about doula training also has increased. Founded in 1992, DONA has grown from a charter membership of 30 to its present size of more than 2,000. Although doulas are not required to be nurses, many of the individuals who contact DONA are labor and delivery nurses. They express frustration in their inability to provide emotional support for labor patients because of reduced staffing, emphasis on technical tasks, and documentation requirements. By working as independent doulas, nurses can provide the needed supportive care.

Many factors have affected the availability of professional nurses for supportive care at the bedside. Down-sizing of professional nursing staff as a result of health care reform in the last decade has affected the number of nurses in birthing units across the nation. This has affected available time that nurses have to provide labor support. McNiven, Hodnett, and O'Brien-Pallas (1992) found that obstetric nurses spent 9.9% of their time providing support to laboring women. Gagnon and Waghorn (1996) reported that 6.1% of a nurse's time at a hospital in Montreal was spent in supportive care. These findings suggest that nurses and hospital administrators must examine how nurses spend their time and develop strategies to maximize the time nurses spend at the bedside providing supportive care.

Further study on the implications of professional versus nonprofessional labor support as it relates to improving patient care and cost is needed (Hodnett, 1998). Doulas, montrices, or professional labor and delivery nurses all can provide labor support. However, it is the education and clinical skills required to assess and intervene quickly when maternal or fetal health status changes that positions the professional nurse as valuable to the laboring woman. Presence at the bedside also enables the professional nurse to remain knowledgeable enough about the patient's health status to collaborate with the attending physician in clinical decision making. In addition, this presence can facilitate advocacy for the patient with other members of the health care team.

Implementing the Guidelines

Each care setting in which a research utilization project is started or new guidelines or protocols are initiated is unique. A universal "cook book" implementation plan would not be useful. Instead, the process for adopting (and evaluating) specific guidelines must be tailored to the individual setting.

A first step involves asking the following questions:

- How will hospital organization affect the process?
- Which colleagues are involved in the process and how are they involved?
- How will the nursing staff be introduced to the protocol?
- What is an acceptable timetable for full implementation?
- For second stage labor protocols, how will the overlap with the medical aspects of care be addressed? (Mayberry, 1994, p.173).

These questions can assist the nurse to identify barriers and facilitators to the implementation of the guidelines. Strategies can then be developed to minimize the barriers and maximize the facilitators. Next, a plan with a time line should be made. An outline for an implementation plan could be similar to the phases of the AWHONN research utilization project: a) hospital support; b) protocol introduction/education; c) protocol implementation/evaluation; and d) local dissemination.

Collaboration with Physicians

The Research Utilization Project on Second Stage Labor Management reinforced the significance of professional nurses in supporting and managing labor. At some sites, physicians were supportive of the changes. The project provided opportunity for increased dialogue among the nurses and physicians. Anesthesia personnel revised their epidural dosage protocols and began to administer dosages based on "the needs of the individual during the second stage of labor" (Niesen & Quirk, 1997, p. 715). However, many site coordinators reported physician resistance to the changes. This led to contradictory instructions to patients during the second stage. For example, a physician would instruct the patient to "hold your breath, count to 10 and push as hard as you can" when the nurse had instructed her to use spontaneous exhalatory (open glottis) bearing down. Contradictory instructions, especially at a stressful time such as the second stage of labor, can undermine the confidence of the woman and her support person in the health care provided. They may become confused about whose instructions to follow.

Findings also showed that physicians often were concerned about the risks of spontaneous pushing in relation to lengthening the second stage. Recognizing that women are at a higher risk for an operative delivery when the second stage is considered to be prolonged, some nurses delayed telling the physicians about a woman's cervical status to delay onset of pushing instructions and, therefore, "buy time" in labor. This example of disparity in clinical practice between nurses and physicians exemplifies a barrier to implementing evidence-based patient care for second stage labor. Increased collaboration and efforts toward more open communication are key to removing this type of barrier.

"Collaboration, a relationship of interdependence, requires the recognition of complementary roles" (Fagin, 1992, p. 354). Nurses and physicians have interdependent, complementary roles in labor management. Once a collaborative environment is established, communication about establishing, implementing, and continually evaluating evidence-based practice protocols and guidelines may be instituted. Researchers have found that patient morbidity and mortality decrease in clinical settings in which "nurse-physician professional collegiality and respectful communication" is evident (Forte, 1997).

Collaboration with Labor and Delivery Nurses

The Research Utilization Project on Second Stage Labor Management demonstrated the challenges that arise during change. During the research utilization process, resistance to change was not only evident with physicians, but also was exhibited by nurses. Some nurses were comfortable with previous practices and chose not to participate in the project. Other nurses had difficulty sustaining the change and would return to prior practices, such as instructing mothers to push by holding their breath or using recumbent positions (Niesen & Quirk, 1997).

On the other hand, many nurses were excited about evaluating a protocol directed at nursing practice. These nurses often were the cheerleaders for the project. Some expressed relief that they were finally given permission to use practices they knew would benefit the mother and fetus (Niesen & Quirk, 1997). Dilemmas can occur when nursing staff are not in sync with each other when caring for the same mother. The patient may receive conflicting instructions. Opportunities for improving the exchange of patient data among labor and delivery nurses are recommended.

Nurses also should be aware that their care during labor may effect the cesarean birth rate. Radin, Harmon, and Hanson (1993) studied the cesarean section rates of healthy nulliparous patients in spontaneous labor cared for labor and delivery nurses at a large nonprofit hospital. Large differences in cesarean sections rates were found among the nurses: the lowest quintile was 4.9%; the highest, 19%. The differences in cesarean rates could not be explained by "maternal age and gravidity, attendance of mother at childbirth class, insurance status, reliance on public assistance, physician who attended labor, use of epidural anesthesia, augmentation of labor, dilation when the nurse assumed care, infant weight or gestational age." (Radin, Harmon, & Hanson, 1993, p. 14).

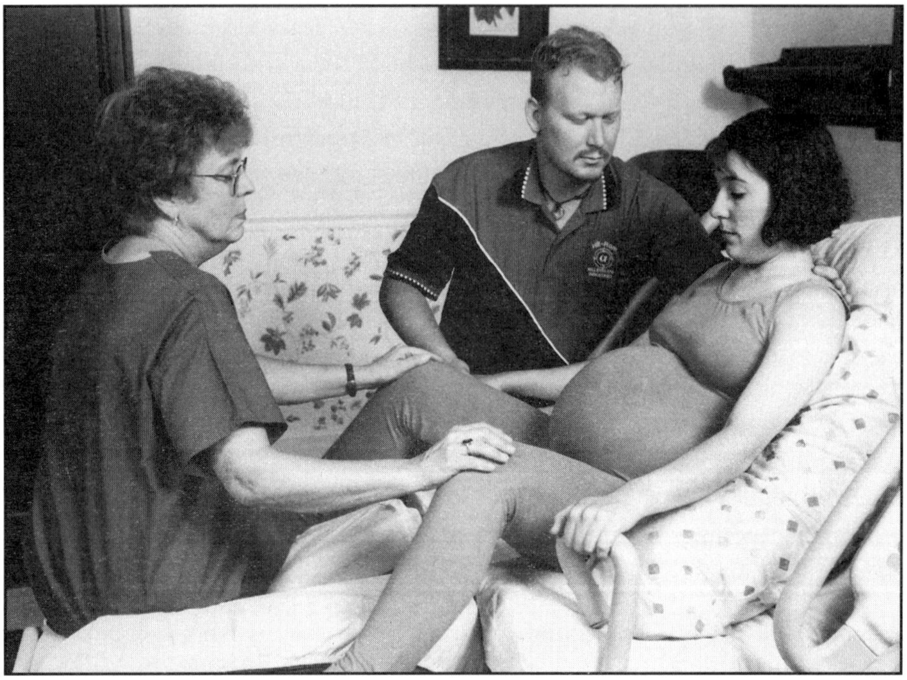

Nurse supporting laboring woman and her significant other during labor.
Photograph compliments of Hill-Rom Company, Inc.

Collaboration with Nurse-Midwives

Collaboration with nurse-midwives also is needed. The philosophical tenet of the nurse-midwifery profession generally is that of advocacy for normalcy. Normalcy, according to Scoggin (1996) is defined as "the nurse-midwife's fundamental belief that a woman's biological and physiological processes are natural and normal" (p. 42). In addition, nurse-midwives recognize the uniqueness of each labor and birth. They tend not to make decisions by the clock or require "...that women labor within the context of rigid rules that constrain her physiologic state or that undermine her confidence..." (Roberts & Woolley, 1996, p. 421). Because labor norms are valued by nurse-midwives along broad parameters, an understanding of the wide variation in labor supports the philosophy of tolerance, rather than intervention in most situations.

Nurse-midwives tend to use fewer interventions and less technology than other obstetric providers. Rosenblatt et al. (1997) compared differences in the intrapartum care of low risk women provided by obstetricians, family practitioners, and certified nurse-midwives. Pregnant women in urban areas throughout Washington state were included. Biologic, as well as sociodemographic differences, were controlled. Birth outcomes were found to be similar for all groups. Statistically significant differences were found related to the number of interventions during the management of the intrapartum period. Specifically, nurse-midwives were less likely to a) induce or augment labor; b) use continuous electronic fetal monitoring; c) administer epidural anesthesia; or d) perform episiotomies. Rosenblatt et al. concluded

> Taken in its totality, this body of knowledge suggests that the approach to low-risk obstetrics as used in the real world by midwives has significant advantage for patients. From a policy perspective, it might be possible to extend the application of this knowledge

by expanding the proportion of deliveries attended by midwives or by transferring some of the skills and philosophy that undergird midwifery to the physicians who practice obstetrics. (Rosenblatt et al., 1997, p. 350)

Collaboration with Childbirth Educators

Although the purpose of the Research Utilization Project on Second Stage Labor Management was to study implementation of intrapartum practices, as the process advanced, other factors that affected the implementation came to light. One such factor was childbirth education. Site coordinator's reports indicated that childbirth education was important to the success of the implementation of intrapartum practices. The stimulus for the site coordinators' observations about childbirth education was the project guideline stating, "All pregnant women should receive information prenatally on the benefits of upright positions for second stage prior to labor." Some site coordinators noted no difficulties with this guideline because a majority of their patients attended childbirth classes that included the suggested content. However, an equal number of site coordinators reported difficulty. The reasons noted for not achieving the objective of this guideline fell into two categories. The first category included barriers to attending childbirth classes. The second category involved a discrepancy between content taught in childbirth classes and actual practices on the labor and delivery unit.

Barriers to Childbirth Education

Location of class, class schedules, lack of child care for older siblings, lack of time to attend, transportation, and cost of childbirth classes are examples of access barriers. An example of a barrier to seeking childbirth education is a woman's lack of awareness of her right to influence, understand, and be involved in her intrapartum care and outcome. A woman's perception that she is not part of a group and, therefore, will not be accepted, also is a barrier to seeking education. Learning barriers may be related to low literacy or language differences. One or a combination of these barriers may be the reason groups such as immigrants; certain ethnic groups (Williams, 1996); and women in high-risk populations, such as teenagers, single women, or substance-abusing women traditionally have low attendance in childbirth classes.

Another access issue is tied to a trend toward discouraging women likely to receive regional analgesia, such as epidurals, from participating in childbirth classes. This advice is based on the assumption that women who choose epidural analgesia will not need the type of classes that provide strategies for coping with labor. This trend puts women at a disadvantage in terms of being prepared for childbirth. It is recommended that, instead, childbirth educators consider providing more content about regional analgesia and encourage these women to participate in childbirth education. Content should acknowledge the extent of pain relief to be expected with epidural analgesia. Potential side effects associated with epidural analgesia, such as prolonged labor and an increased risk for cesarean delivery, also should be covered.

Each community and health care setting should identify barriers for their populations, determine individual solutions, and develop approaches for increasing participation in childbirth education. Childbirth educators can improve access by collaborating with employers to ensure that childbirth education is a component of health care benefit packages for employees. The March of Dimes publication, *Healthy Babies, Healthy Business: An Employer's Guidebook on Improving Maternal and Infant Health* (1993) that was developed for benefits specialists may be helpful. This manual outlines elements of a comprehensive maternal-child benefits package that includes childbirth education classes and outlines a staged approach for adopting the elements into company benefits programs.

Population specific classes for certain groups, such as immigrants, teenagers, substance-abusing women, and various cultural groups may increase the number of prepared women. For example, in New York City, an existing program was modified for teenagers and substance-abusing women. Changes were made in the course content and in class scheduling to appeal to these groups (Carrington et al., 1994). In Canada, non-traditional classes for First Nation participants (referred to as Native Americans in the United States) involve story-telling and oral histories told by the respected elders and other women of the communities.

Discrepancy Between Content in Childbirth Education Classes and Practices on the Labor and Delivery Unit

Even when childbirth education is available to women who readily participate, a discrepancy may exist between content taught versus actual practice on a particular labor and delivery unit. This discrepancy is particularly true regarding content about second stage labor. According to the site coordinators, women or couples receive preparation for coping in labor, such as ambulation, position changes, and alternative pushing techniques, but are then denied these options. The women or couples often were told, "That isn't how we do it here." For example, in a childbirth class at one of the sites, women were taught to use "short, grunty pushes" when a premature urge to bear down with contractions occurs; however, during labor, women were instructed to "pant" in response.

Numerous childbirth education programs and instructors further contribute to this dichotomy. Labor and delivery nurses said that because of the variety of programs, it is difficult to know what is actually taught in classes. Similarly, when classes consist of couples delivering in a variety of hospitals and under the care of differing providers, childbirth educators have difficulty knowing specific practices of each setting. Childbirth educators are confronted with a dilemma about what to teach their clients. For example, although the practice of limiting the length of second stage labor is changing, not all settings have adopted the change.

Finally, perhaps more labor and delivery nurses with an interest in childbirth education should be encouraged to seek certification as childbirth educators. A finding from the research utilization project was that only 12.2% of the labor and delivery nurses at the participating hospitals were childbirth educators. It is difficult to assess to what extent this percentage represents a possible decline in numbers of nurses providing childbirth education or whether this perceived decline has played a role in the incongruity between consumer education and actual practice.

Communication among childbirth educators and intrapartum care providers is key to increasing access and closing the gap between childbirth education content and intrapartum practices. Such communication may increase the knowledge of evidence-based practice for all involved. For example, a college located near one of the RU sites that sponsors a childbirth education program created an advisory board whose members include consumers, representatives from local hospitals, childbirth educators, public health nurses, and physicians. The board meets regularly throughout the year to discuss issues, plan strategies, and provide input on curriculum changes. Additionally, one of the Research Utilization Project hospital sites conducts an annual meeting for nurses and local childbirth educators. Policy updates are provided, and solutions for current issues are discussed. At these meetings, the childbirth educators share their own ideas and concerns as well as those of consumers.

Future of Childbirth Education

Leaders in the field of childbirth education are examining the content and timing of childbirth education. According to Constance Castor, president of the Council for Childbirth Education Specialists Inc., there is a movement away from the prescribed education content of the 1960s and 1970s to an emphasis on strengthening a sense of mastery (personal communication, August 1996). Gaining mastery involves developing an understanding of the interconnectedness of body and mind and the benefits that come from shaping these connections. To further this goal, childbirth education will need to become more individualized and begin during the 1st trimester.

Beginning in the 1st trimester, women should be educated on the use of muscle relaxation exercises and progressive body awareness strategies. These strategies can be taught in conjunction with muscle strengthening exercises. Tupler (1996) recommended, for example, that specific exercises designed to prepare women for squatting positions used in the second stage of labor should be started in early pregnancy.

Recognition of and increased responsiveness to internal and external cues also is essential. Therefore, it would not be necessary, for example, "to teach women how to push" during labor if they are taught to listen to their own bodies (personal communication, Constance Castor, August 1996). The benefits of upright positioning during labor should receive a stronger emphasis, and more in-depth information on the range of pain relief options, particularly epidural analgesia, should be addressed. Attention to the benefits and potential adverse effects of narcotics and regional analgesia should be provided before the actual labor and delivery. An understanding of the risks for cesarean delivery also is important content.

Finally, assisting women to develop assessment and negotiation skills to assess their care and make decisions collaboratively with their health care providers should be included. Doing so strengthens the premise that the childbearing period is an opportune time to contribute to the woman's ability to advocate for her own health. Assessment and negotiation skills are essential to women throughout their lives as they plan and direct care for themselves and their families.

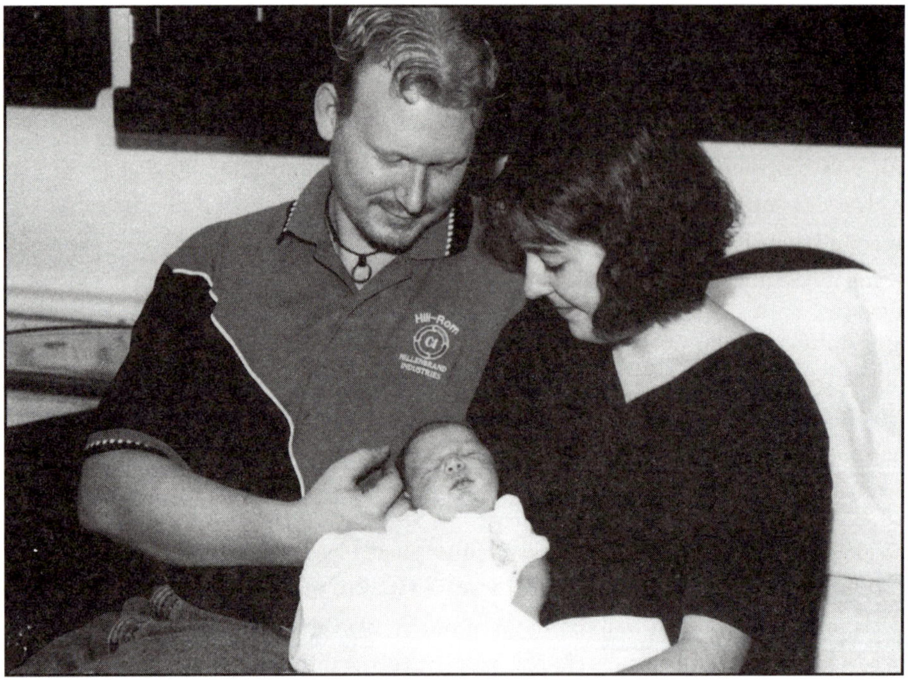

Photograph compliments of Hill-Rom Company, Inc.

Conclusion

As with many areas of health care; new trends in therapies and advances in technology have positively influenced the philosophy and conduct of patient care. However, new dilemmas sometimes are created by these same trends and advances. This has been the case with hospital-based care of women in labor, particularly during the second stage. Nurses and physicians have a responsibility to question the rationale for all interventions and evaluate the efficacy of research findings that apply in the labor and delivery setting. For this to happen, increased efforts toward interdisciplinary collaboration among nurses; physicians; nurse-midwives; childbirth educators; and pregnant women, as informed consumers of this care, will continue to be important.

References

Aderhold, K.J., & Roberts, J.E. (1991). Phases of second stage labor. *Journal of Nurse Midwifery,* 36(15), 267–275.

Albers, L.L., Schiff, M., & Gorwoda, J.G. (1996). The length of active labor in normal pregnancies. *Obstetrics and Gynecology,* 87, 355–359.

Aldrich, C.J., D'Antona, D., Spencer, J.A., Wyatt, J.S., Peebles, D.M., Delpy, D.T., & Reynolds, E.O. (1995). The effect of maternal pushing on fetal cerebral oxygenation and blood volume during the second stage of labour. *British Journal of Obstetrics and Gynaecology,* 102, 448–453.

Allen, R.E., Hosker, G.L., Smith, A.R.B., & Warrell, D.W. (1990). Pelvic floor damage and childbirth: A neurophysiological study. *British Journal of Obstetrics and Gynaecology,* 97, 770–779.

American College of Obstetricians and Gynecologists. (1994). Operative vaginal delivery *(ACOG Technical Bulletin #196),* Washington, DC: Author.

Barnett, M. M., & Humenick, S.S. (1982). Infant outcome in relation to second stage labor pushing method. *Birth,* 9, 221–229.

Benyon, C.L. (1957). The normal second stage of labour: A plea for reform in its conduct. *Journal of Obstetrics and Gynecology of the British Empire,* 64, 815–820.

Breen, T.W., Shapiro, T., Glass, B., Foster-Payne, D., & Oriol, N.E. (1993). Epidual anesthesia for labor in an ambulatory patient. *Anesthesia and Analgesia,* 77, 919–924.

Caldeyro-Barcia, R. (1979). The influence of maternal bearing-down efforts during second stage on fetal well-being. *Birth and the Family Journal,* 6, 17–21.

Carrington, B.W., Loftman, P.O., Boucher, E., Irish, G., Piniaz, D.K., & Mitchell, J.L. (1994). Modifying a childbirth education curriculum for two specific populations. Inner-city adolescents and substance-using women. *Journal of Nurse-Midwifery,* 39, 312–320.

Chalmers, I., Enkin, M., & Keirse, M.J.N.C. (1989). *Effective care in pregnancy and childbirth.* London: Oxford University Press.

Cohen, W.R. (1977). Influence of the duration of second stage labor on perinatal outcome and puerperal morbidity. *Obstetrics and Gynecology,* 49, 266–269.

Cosner, K.R., & deJong, E. (1993). Physiologic second-stage labor. *MCN: American Journal of Maternal Child Nursing,* 18(1), 38–43.

de Jong, P.R., Johanson, R.B., Baxen, P., Adrians, V.D., van der Westhuisen, S., & Jones, P.W. (1997). Randomised trial comparing the upright and supine positions for the second stage of labour. *British Journal of Obstetrics & Gynaecology,* 104, 567–571.

Dewan, D.M., & Cohen, S.E. (1994). Epidural analgesia and the incidence of cesarean section: Time for a closer look. *Anesthesiology,* 80, 1189–1192

Dundes, L. (1987). The evolution of maternal birthing position. *American Journal of Public Health,* 77, 636–641.

Eddleston, J.M., Holland, J.J., Griffin, R.P., Corbett, A., Horsman, E.L., & Reynolds, F. (1996). A double-blind comparison of 0.25% ripovacaine and 0.25% bupivacine for extradural analgesia in labour. *British Journal of Anaesthesia,* 76 (1), 66–71.

Enkin, M., Keirse, M.J.N.C., Renfrew, M., & Neilson, J. (1995). *A guide to effective care in pregnancy and childbirth (2nd ed.).* New York: Oxford University Press.

Executive Communications, Inc. (1993). Second stage labor nursing management: *Practice issues.* Dallas: TX (Video).

Davies, J. & Renning, E.L. (1964). The birth canal: Practical applications. *Medical Times,* 92(1), 75–86.

Fagin, C.M. (1992). Collaboration between nurses and physicians: No longer a choice. *Academic Medicine,* 67, 295–303.

Flamm, B.L., Berwick, D.M., & Kabcenell, A. (1998). Reducing cesarean section rates safely: Lessons from a "breakthrough series" collaborative. *Birth,* 25(2), 117–124.

Flynn, A.M., Kelly, J., Hollins, G., & Lynch, P.F. (1978). Ambulation in labour. *British Medical Journal,* 2(6137), 591–593.

Forte, P.S. (1997). The high cost of conflict. *Nursing Economics,* 15, 119–123.

Friedman, E.A. (1954). The graphic analysis of labor. *American Journal of Obstetrics and Gynecology,* 68, 1568–1575.

Funk, S.G., Tornquist, E.M., & Champagne, M.T. (1995). Barriers and facilitators of research utilization: An integrative review. *Nursing Clinics of North America,* 30, 395–407.

Gagnon, A.J., & Waghorn, K. (1996). Supportive care by maternity nurses: A work sampling study in an intrapartum unit. *Birth,* 23, 1–6.

Gardosi, J., Sylvester, S., & Lynch, C.B. (1989). Alternative positions in the second stage of labor: A randomized trial. B*ritish Journal of Obstetrics & Gynecology,* 96(11), 1290–1296.

Gennaro, S. (1994). Research utilization: An overview. *Journal of Obstetric, Gynecologic, and Neonatal Nursing,* 23, 313–319.

Gleeson, N.C., & Griffith, A. P. (1991). The management of second stage of labour in primiparae with epidural analgesia. *British Journal of Clinical Practice,* 45, 90–91.

Golay, J., Vedam, S., & Sorger, L. (1993). The squatting position for the second stage of labor: Effects on labor and on maternal and fetal well-being. *Birth,* 20, 73–78.

Grimes, D.A. (1995). Introducing evidence-based medicine into a department of obstetrics and gynecology. *Obstetrics and Gynecology,* 86, 451–457.

Gupta, J.K., Brayshaw, E.M., & Lilford, R.J. (1989). An experiment of squatting birth. *European Journal of Obstetrics, Gynecology and Reproductive Biology,* 30, 217–220.

Handa, V.L., Harris, T.A., & Ostergard, D.R. (1996). Protecting the pelvic floor: Obstetric management to prevent incontinence and pelvic organ prolapse. *Obstetrics & Gynecology,* 88, 470–478.

Hansen, S.L., & Clark, S. L. (1996). Rest and descend vs. pushing with epidural anesthesia in the 2nd stage of labor. *American Journal of Obstetrics and Gynecology,* 174, 479.

Hodnett, E. (1996). Nursing support of the laboring woman. *Journal of Obstetric, Gynecologic, and Neonatal Nursing,* 25, 257–264.

Hodnett, E.D. (1998). *Support from caregivers during childbirth (Cochrane Review).* In: The Cochrane Library, Issue 3. Oxford: Update Software.

Hodnett, E.D., & Osborn, R.W. (1989). A randomized trial of the effects of monitrice support during labor: Mothers' views two to four weeks postpartum. *Birth,* 16, 177–183.

Holland, R.L., & Smith, D.A. (1989). Management of the second stage of labor: A review (Part II). Maternal positioning as it relates to the management of the second stage of labor is reviewed. *South Dakota Journal of Medicine,* 42 (6), 5–8.

Hordnes, K., & Bergsjo, P. (1993). Severe lacerations after childbirth. *Acta Obstetricia et Gynecologica Scandinavica,* 72, 413–422.

Humphrey, M., Hounslow, D., Morgan, S., & Wood, C. (1973). The influence of maternal posture at birth on the fetus. *Journal of Obstetrics annd Gynecology of the British Commonwealth,* 80, 1075–1080.

Johnson, N., Johnson, V.A., & Gupta, J.K. (1991). Maternal positions during labor. *Obstetrical and Gynecological Survey,* 46(7), 428–434.

Leveno, K.J., Cunningham, F.G., Nelson, S., Roark, M., Williams, M.L., Guzick, D., Dowling, S., Rosenfeld, C.R., & Buckley, A. (1986). A prospective comparison of selective and universal electronic fetal monitoring in 34,995 pregnancies. *New England Journal of Medicine,* 315, 615–619.

Lieberman, E., Lang, J.M., Cohen, A., D'Agostino, R. Jr., Datta, S., & Frigoletto, F.D. Jr. (1996). Association of epidural analgesia with cesarean delivery in nulliparas. *Obstetrics and Gynecology,* 88 (6), 993–1000.

Lindsey, A.M. (1991). Integrating research and practice. In M.M. Mateo & K.T. Kirchhoff (Eds.), *Conducting and using research in the clinical setting* (pp. 103–104). Baltimore: Williams & Wilkins.

Liu, Y.C. (1974). Effects of an upright position during labor. *American Journal of Nursing,* 74, 2202–2205.

Luthy, D.A., Shy, K.K., van Belle, G., Larson, E.B., Hughes, J.P., Benedetti, T.J., Brown, Z.A., Effer, S., King, J.F., & Stenchever, M.A. (1987). A randomized trial of electronic fetal monitoring in preterm labor. *Obstetrics and Gynecology,* 69, 687–695.

Manyonda, I.T., Shaw, D.E., & Drife, J.0. (1990). The effect of delayed pushing in the second stage of labor with continuous lumbar epidural analgesia. *Acta Obstetricia et Gynecologica Scandinavica,* 69, 291–295.

March of Dimes Birth Defects Foundation. (1993). Healthy babies, healthy business: *An employer's guidebook on improving maternal and infant health.* White Plains, NY: Author.

Maresh, M., Choong, K.H., & Beard, R.W. (1983). Delayed pushing with lumbar epidural analgesia in labour. *British Journal of Obstetrics and Gynaecology,* 90, 623–627.

Mayberry, L. (1994). Intrapartum nursing care: Research into practice. *Journal of Obstetric, Gynecologic, and Neonatal Nursing,* 23, 170–174.

Mayberry, L.J., Gennaro, S., Strange, L., Williams, M., & De, A. (1999). Maternal fatigue: Implications of second stage labor nursing care. *Journal of Obstetric, Gynecologic, and Neonatal Nurses,* 28, 175–181.

Mayberry, L.J., Hammer, R., Kelly, C., True-Driver, B., & De, A. (1998). Use of delayed pushing with epidural anesthesia: Findings from a randomized, controlled trial. *Journal of Perinatology,* 19 (1), 26–30.

Mayberry, L.J., & Strange, L.B. (1997). Strategies for designing a research utilization project with labor and delivery nurses. *Journal of Obstetric, Gynecologic, and Neonatal Nursing,* 26, 701–708.

Mayberry, L., Wood, S., & Held, N. (1993). Second stage labor management: Why can't we progress [oral presentation]. Challenges Beyond Limits. Reno, NV: Association of Women's Health, Obstetric, and Neonatal Nurses.

McClure, J.H. (1996). Ropivacaine. *British Journal of Anaestheia,* 76 (2), 300–307.

McKay, S. (1984). Squatting: An alternate position for the second stage of labor. *MCN: American Journal of Maternal Child Nursing,* 9(3), 181–183.

McKay, S. (1981). Second stage labor: Has tradition replaced safety? *American Journal of Nursing,* 81, 1016–1019.

McKay, S., Barrows, T., & Roberts, J. (1990). Women's views of second stage as assessed by interviews and videotapes. *Birth,* 17(4), 266–273.

McKay, S., & Roberts, J. (1990). Obstetrics by ear: Maternal and caregiver perceptions of the meaning of maternal sound during the second stage of labor. *Journal of Nurse Midwifery,* 35(5), 266–273.

McNiven, P., Hodnett, E., & O' Brien-Pallas, L.L. (1992). Supporting women in labor: A work sampling of the activities of labor and delivery nurses. *Birth,* 19, 3–9.

Medoff-Cooper, B. (1994). Transition of the preterm infant to an open crib. *Journal of Obstetric, Gynecologic, and Neonatal Nursing,* 23, 329–335.

Menticoglou, S.M., Manning, F., Harman, C., & Morrison, I. (1995). Perinatal outcomes in relation to second-stage duration. *American Journal of Obstetrics and Gynecology,* 173, 906–912.

Muir, H.A., Writer, D., Douglas, J., Weeks, S., Gambling, D., & MacArthur, A. (1997). Double blind comparison of epidural ropivacaine 0.25% and bupivacaine 0.25% for the relief of childbirth pain. *Canadian Journal of Anaesthesia,* 44 (6), 599–604.

Niesen, K.M., & Quirk, A.G. (1997). The process for initiating nursing practice changes in the intrapartum: Findings from a multisite research utilization project. *Journal of Obstetric, Gynecologic, and Neonatal Nursing,* 26, 709–717.

Paciornik, M. (1990). Commentary: Arguments against episiotomy and in favor of squatting for birth. *Birth,* 17, 104–105.

Paine, L.L., & Dawkins-Tinker, D. (1992). Affect of maternal bearing down efforts on umbilical cord pH and length of second stage of labor. *Journal of Nurse Midwifery,* 37 (1), 61–63.

Philipsen, T., & Jensen, N.H. (1989). Epidural block or parenteral pethidine as analgesic in labour: A randomized study concerning progress in labour and instrumental deliveries. *European Journal of Obstetrics, Gynecology and Reproductive Biology,* 30, 27–33.

Radin, T.G., Harmon, J.S., & Hanson, D.A. (1993). Nurses'care during labor: Its effect on the cesarean birth rate of healthy, nulliparous women. *Birth,* 20(1), 14–21.

Ramin, S.M., Gambling, D.R., Lucas, M.J., Sharma, S.K., Sidawi, J.E., & Leveno, J.K. (1995). Randomized trial of epidural verses intravenous analgesia during labor. *Obstetrics and Gynecology,* 86, 783–789.

Read, J.A., Miller, F.C., & Paul, R.H. (1981). Randomized trial of ambulation versus oxytocin for labor enhancement: A preliminary report. *American Journal of Obstetrics and Gynecology,* 139, 669–672.

Roberts, J. (1980). Alternative positions for childbirth. Part II: Second stage of labor. *Journal of Nurse Midwifery,* 25(5), 13–19.

Roberts, J.E., Goldstein, S.A., Gruener, J.S., Maggio, M., & Mendez-Bauer, C. (1987). A descriptive analysis of involuntary bearing down efforts during the expulsive phase of labor. *Journal of Obstetric, Gynecologic, and Neonatal Nursing,* 16, 48–55.

Roberts, J.E., Mendez-Bauer, C., & Wodell, D.A. (1983). The effects of maternal positioning on uterine contractility and efficiency, *Birth,* 10(4), 243–249.

Roberts, J., & Woolley, D. (1996). A second look at the second stage of labor. *Journal of Obstetric, Gynecologic, and Neonatal Nursing,* 25, 415–423.

Rosen, M.G., & Dickinson, J.C. (1993). The paradox of electronic fetal monitoring: More data may not enable us to predict or prevent neurologic morbidity. *American Journal of Obstetrics and Gynecology,* 168, 745–751.

Rosenblatt, R.A., Dobie, S.A., Hart, L.G., Schneeweiss, R., Gould, D., Raine, T.R., Benedetti, T.J., Pirani, M.J., & Perrin, E.B. (1997). Interspecialty differences in the obstetric care of low-risk women. *American Journal of Public Health,* 87, 344–351.

Russell, J.G.B. (1982). The rationale of primitive delivery positions. *British Journal of Obstetrics and Gynecology,* 89, 712–715.

Sachs, B.P., Kobelin, C., Castro, M.A., & Frigoletto, F. (1999). The risks of lowering the cesarean-delivery rate. *New England Journal of Medicine,* 340, 57–57.

Sampselle, C.M., & Hines, S. (1999). Spontaneous pushing during birth: Relationship to perineal outcomes. *Journal of Nurse Midwifery,* 44, 36–39.

Sandmire, H.F. (1990). Whither electronic fetal monitoring? *Obstetrics and Gynecology,* 76, 1130–1134.

Schneider, H., Progler, M., Ziegler, W.H., & Huch, R. (1990). Biochemical changes in the mother and the fetus during labor and its significance for the management of the second stage. *International Journal of Gynaecology and Obstetrics,* 31, 117–126.

Scoggin, J. (1996). How nurse-midwives define themselves in relation to nursing, medicine, and midwifery. *Journal of Nurse-Midwifery,* 41, 36–42.

Shermer, R.H., & Raines, D.A. (1997). Positioning during the second stage of labor: Moving back to basics. *Journal of Obstetric, Gynecologic, and Neonatal Nursing,* 26, 727–734.

Simkin, P. (1982). Preparing parents for second stage. *Birth,* 9(4), 229.

Sleep, J., Roberts, J., & Chalmers, I. (1989). Care during the second stage of labor. In I. Chalmers, M. Enkin, & M.J.N.C. Keirse (Eds.), *Effective care in pregnancy and childbirth* (pp. 1129–1144). New York: Oxford University Press.

Sloane, E. (1993). *Biology of women* (3rd ed.). Albany, NY: Delmar.

Society of Obstetricians and Gynaecologists of Canada. (1995). Fetal health surveillance in labor. (SOGC Policy Statement). *Journal SOGC,* 17, 865–901.

Taylor, S.E. (1983). Adjustment to threatening events: A theory of cognitive adaptation. *American Psychologist,* 38, 1161–1173.

Thorp, J.A., Hu, D.H., Albin, R.M., McNitt, J., Meyer, B.A., Cohen, G.R., & Yeast, J.D. (1993). The effect of intrapartum epidural analgesia on nulliparous labor: A randomized, controlled, prospective trial. *American Journal of Obstetrics and Gynecology,* 169, 851–858.

Tupler, J. (1996). *Maternal fitness: Preparing for the marathon of labor.* New York: Simon and Schuster.

Vause, S., Congdon, H.M., & Thornton, J. G. (1998). Immediate and delayed pushing in the second stage of labour for nulliparous women with epidural analgesia: A randomized controlled trial. *British Journal of Obstetrics and Gynaecology,* 105, 186–188.

Williams, L.S. (1996). Study of new mothers looks at language and cultural barriers facing immigrant women. *CMAJ,* 154, 1563–1564.

Wittels, B. (1991). Does epidural anesthesia affect the course of labor and delivery? *Seminars in Perinatology,* 15, 358–367.

Youngstrom, P.C., Baker, S.W., & Miller, J.L. Epidurals redefined in analgesia and anesthesia: A distinction with a difference. *Journal of Obstetric, Gynecologic, and Neonatal Nurses,* 25, 350–354.

Yun, E.M., Meadows, W., & Santos, A.C. (1998). New amide local anesthetics for obstetric use. In A. Ross (Ed.), *Bailliere's Clinical Obstetrics and Gynaecology,* 12 (3), 461–471.

Zhang, J., Bernasko, J.W., Leybovich, E., Fahs, M., & Hatch, M.C. (1996) Continuous labor support from labor attendant for primiparous women: A meta anaylsis. *Obstetrics and Gynecology,* 88, 739–744.

Second Stage Labor Management: Promotion of Evidence-Based Practice and a Collaborative Approach to Patient Care

Goal: To inform nurses about research-based interdisciplinary strategies for the care of women during the second stage of labor to facilitate optimal maternal/neonatal outcomes.

Objectives:

- Describe the process for promoting evidence-based practices toward improving the quality of second stage labor care for women.
- Delineate the physiologic basis for the use of upright positioning and self-regulating bearing down or "pushing" during second stage labor.
- Discuss the major practice issues associated with the need to increase collaboration among nurses, physicians, and childbirth educators when providing care for women in labor and delivery.

Post Test Questions

1. An increased risk for cesarean delivery has been associated with care practices used during the second stage of labor in many hospitals throughout the United States and Canada.
   A. True
   B. False
2. Current ACOG recommendations state that the duration of second stage labor should:
   A. Be limited to 2 hours or less.
   B. Be individualized according to maternal/fetal status parameters.
   C. Not be a practice issue when women receive epidural analgesia.
3. Use of labor curve norms to dictate the absolute duration of second stage labor has been challenged based on findings from reported research studies during the last decade.
   A. True
   B. False
4. Potential outcomes associated with directed, strong, and sustained "pushing" efforts during the second stage of labor include:
   A. A higher risk for both short and long-term pelvic floor damage.
   B. Less maternal intrapartum and postpartum fatigue.
   C. A lower risk for the development of short-term fetal hypoxia.
5. Which of the following maternal positions for second stage labor may contribute to an increased incidence of episiotomy and perineal lacerations?
   A. Squatting.
   B. Sitting on the bedside.
   C. Lithotomy.
6. The use of upright positions during second stage labor has been associated with:
   A. A higher incidence of episiotomy and perineal lacerations.
   B. An increased risk for fetal heart rate decelerations.
   C. Enhanced fetal descent due to improved fetal/pelvic alignment and the positive effects of gravity.
7. A recommended position for second stage labor is:
   A. Lithotomy
   B. Semi-Fowlers
   C. Squatting
8. Epidural analgesia during second stage labor:
   A. Is always a contraindication to the use of upright positioning.
   B. Has been associated with an increased risk for cesarean delivery in reported research studies.
   C. Is recommended only for multiparous women following a prolonged first stage of labor.

Second Stage Labor Management

9. Initiation of "pushing" efforts by women during the second stage should be encouraged following:
   A. Artificial rupture of membranes.
   B. Complete cervical dilation accompanied by the maternal urge to bear down.
   C. Complete cervical dilation with fetal stations of -2 to 0, regardless of the presence of the urge to "push".
10. The negative fetal consequences associated with prolonged labors may be due to:
    A. Sustained pushing efforts and maternal breath-holding across a lengthy period of time.
    B. The use of "open glottis" bearing down efforts.
    C. Ferguson's reflex.
11. Efforts to reduce unnecessary cesarean deliveries can be enhanced through which of the following strategies?
    A. Less childbirth education for those women receiving epidural analgesia.
    B. More frequent use of routine electronic fetal heart rate monitoring.
    C. Intensified collaboration between physicians and nurses to individualize research-based care during second stage labor.
12. Which of the following should **not** continue to be an important focus of childbirth education?
    A. Knowledge of body awareness cues and responsiveness beginning in the first trimester.
    B. Learning specific techniques for pushing beginning in the third trimester.
    C. Development of assessment and negotiation skills to enhance collaborative decisionmaking with health care providers.
13. Which of the following is **not** a common discrepancy between childbirth education content and the actual practices that are implemented on many labor and delivery units?
    A. Significance of ambulation and position changes during labor.
    B. Alternative "pushing" options to closed-glottis pushing.
    C. Labor support comfort measures for mother and fathers.
14. Which of the following has **not** been reported as a possible barrier to research utilization by nurses?
    A. Inadequate staffing and limited institutional support.
    B. Increased dialogue about clinical research findings between researchers and clinicians.
    C. Difficulty in finding relevant clinical research with practice implications.
15. The presence of continuous labor support for women:
    A. Is not necessary if anesthesiologists are available to monitor epidural dosage levels.
    B. Has been associated with positive maternal and neonatal outcomes.
    C. Increases the risk for maternal intrapartum complications.
16. Barriers to receiving childbirth education that have been identified include which of the following?
    A. Lack of encouragement by health care providers when epidural analgesia is available.
    B. Increasing numbers of labor and delivery nurses involved in childbirth education.
    C. Use of community advisory boards to discuss curriculum issues.
17. Criteria for nurses to use in evaluating whether research findings are ready for clinical application do **not** include which of the following?
    A. Scientific merit.
    B. Feasibility established in terms of cost-benefit advantages.
    C. Immediate on-unit medical staff acceptance.
18. Professional nursing support in labor is recommended because:
    A. Their education and clinical skills afford the ability to intervene quickly when maternal/fetal health status changes.
    B. Most women should be confined to bed during second stage labor.
    C. All women require constant surveillance of normal fetal heart rate patterns.

Second Stage
Labor Management

Participant Evaluation Form

TIME:

Time required to read and study the content and complete the posttest:

_________ minutes.

LEARNING OBJECTIVES:

Using a scale of 1 (not effective) through 5 (highly effective) please rate, by circling a number, how effectively the independent study enabled you to meet each of the following objectives:

	Not Effective				Highly Effective
1. Describe the process for promoting evidence-based practices toward improving the quality of second stage labor care for women.	1	2	3	4	5
2. Delineate the physiologic basis for the use of upright positioning and self-regulating bearing down or "pushing" during second stage labor.	1	2	3	4	5
3. Discuss the major practice issues associated with the need to increase collaboration among nurses, physicians, and childbirth educators when providing care for women in labor and delivery.	1	2	3	4	5

Second Stage Labor Management

OVERALL RATINGS:

Using a rating scale of 1 (poor) through 5 (excellent), please rate the following areas:

	Poor				Excellent
1. Relationship of objectives to overall purpose/goal	1	2	3	4	5
2. Timeliness of content	1	2	3	4	5
3. Usefulness of content to clinical practice	1	2	3	4	5
4. Effectiveness as a learning resource	1	2	3	4	5

Other comments and suggestions:

____

____

____

____

Continuing Education Credit Application Form

2.3 contact hours of CE credit for this program may be earned until 6/30/02.

INSTRUCTIONS

1. After reading and studying the educational module, take the posttest and indicate your answers on the Posttest Answers section of this form.
2. Complete the Participant Evaluation Form and this Application Form. Make a copy of these forms and your posttest answers for your records.
3. Mail the Participant Evaluation Form and the Application Form, along with a check for $10 (AWHONN member) or $20 (non-AWHONN member) to: AWHONN, Independent Study, 2000 L Street, NW, Suite 740, Washington, DC 20036.
4. Certificates will be issued to participants upon receipt of the completed evaluation form, application, and processing fee. A copy of the posttest answers will be mailed with each certificate for self-scoring of the posttest.
5. Questions regarding this program or the process of applying for CE credit should be directed to:

   Education Programs Coordinator
   AWHONN
   2000 L Street, NW, Suite 740
   Washington, DC 20036
   Telephone: (202) 261-2417

Second Stage
Labor Management

Checks should be made payable to AWHONN.

AWHONN is accredited as a provider of continuing education in nursing by the American Nurses Credentialing Center's Commission on Accreditation and holds California and Alabama BRN numbers. California CE provider #BRN00580; Alabama Board of Nursing Provider #ABNP0058

NOTE: AWHOHNN contact hour credit does not imply approval or endorsement of any product(s).

Second Stage Labor Management: Promotion of Evidence-Based Practice and a Collaborative Approach to Patient Care

I have enclosed a check or money order for $______, payable to AWHONN. (Payment must be included for your examination to be processed.)

NAME______________________________

STREET______________________________

ADDRESS______________________________

CITY____________________ STATE__________ ZIP________

DAYTIME PHONE NO.______________________________

POSTTEST ANSWERS

Please write the letter of the correct answer in the space below:

1. ______	4. ______	7. ______	10. ______	13. ______	16. ______
2. ______	5. ______	8. ______	11. ______	14. ______	17. ______
3. ______	6. ______	9. ______	12. ______	15. ______	18. ______